# Understanding the
# Mammography Controversy

# Understanding the Mammography Controversy

## SCIENCE, POLITICS, AND BREAST CANCER SCREENING

Madelon L. Finkel

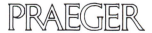
PRAEGER

Westport, Connecticut
London

**Library of Congress Cataloging-in-Publication Data**

Finkel, Madelon Lubin, 1949–
    Understanding the mammography controversy : science, politics, and breast cancer
screening / Madelon L. Finkel.
        p. cm.
    Includes bibliographical references and index.
    ISBN 0–275–98188–6 (alk. paper)
    1. Breast—Cancer—Diagnosis—Evaluation.   2. Medical screening—Evaluation.
    3. Breast—Cancer—Risk factors.   4. Breast—Radiography.   I. Title.
    RA645.C3F54 2005
    616.99'449075—dc22        2004028037

British Library Cataloguing in Publication Data is available.

Library of Congress Catalog Card Number: 2004028037
ISBN: 0–275–98188–6

First published in 2005

Praeger Publishers, 88 Post Road West, Westport, CT 06881
An imprint of Greenwood Publishing Group, Inc.
www.praeger.com

Printed in the United States of America

The paper used in this book complies with the
Permanent Paper Standard issued by the National
Information Standards Organization (Z39.48–1984).

10 9 8 7 6 5 4 3 2 1

To my mother, Lorraine Lubin, who never
let her breast cancer get in the way
of enjoying and living her life to its fullest
and
To my daughter, Rebecca Finkel

# Contents

# Acknowledgment

Many thanks to William Feldman, who spent a summer researching the topic and who rapidly learned how confusing epidemiological research can be. Thanks also to David Hyman, who as a first-year medical student at the Weill Medical College of Cornell University, spent a summer researching communication issues in the doctor–patient relationship. Their assistance, hard work, and sense of humor are greatly appreciated. Sincere thanks to Marsha Gordon who shared her thoughts, feelings, and fears about her breast cancer with me. She is happily in remission. Many thanks to colleague Ellen Warshauer for her insightful comments on the first draft of the book manuscript.

CHAPTER 1

# The Female Breast

Over the centuries, the female breast has been depicted as a symbol of many things including fertility, liberty (political symbol of liberty in the French Revolution, for example), eroticism, obsession (as in Freud's obsession), and female liberation. Breasts are depicted in paintings, sculptures, and drawings. Psychiatrists and psychologists, religious leaders, advertisers, and pornographers have either rhapsodized or vilified the female breast; and, males, for eons, have fantasized about this part of the female body. Ever-changing fashion styles have gyrated from covering up the breast, to seductively exposing a significant portion of the breast, to "letting it all hang out." But, from a historical view, "obsession" with the female breast is a fairly recent phenomenon.

The fascination with the female breast seems to transcend time and place. Of course there are widespread cultural differences in attitudes about female breasts and the role they play in sexual attraction. In some developing societies, females rarely cover their breasts; in most other places in the world, conventional dress and social mores dictate that a woman's breasts are not exposed. The European attitudes about female breasts, covered or uncovered, are quite different than American attitudes. In Europe, going topless at the beach is quite accepted and considered normal. In the United States, public bathing places have laws against such display. At the other end of the spectrum, in the Muslim countries of the Middle East, women of certain sects are not allowed to show any part of their body in public. Other sects permit the woman to show her face, but the rest of her body is covered.

## THE FEMALE BREAST AS VIEWED THROUGH HISTORY

The breast is depicted in Egyptian papyri dating from the eighteenth dynasty, and in the second century BCE, the first well-known written work on human sexuality, the Kama Sutra, made reference to breasts. For the most part, however, the female breast has been depicted in other forms of visual art, including sculpture, painting, and drawing. In ancient Egyptian hieroglyphics, for example, the Egyptian goddess Isis is depicted nursing a pharaoh. Although women at that time accented their breasts with cosmetics and exotic scents, there is little evidence to indicate that the female breast was depicted or perceived as a sexual magnet for males.

Early Christian art tended to portray females with one or both breasts uncovered. Marilyn Yalom, author of A History of the Breast, writes that the breast pre-1400, especially, was viewed as a sacred object.[1] The image of the nurturing Madonna of fourteenth-century Italy, for example, was not considered lewd or indecent at the time. The Sistine Chapel, too, is adorned with paintings of women with one or both breasts uncovered as well as scenes of nudity. These religious paintings depict the breast in a maternal form, a nursing Madonna, and the like. During the Renaissance, a more sensual, even erotic, image of the female breast was portrayed in art. The voluptuous woman with breasts bulging out of her garments is a familiar sight in paintings of the time.

Throughout the ages, fashion both served to accentuate a woman's breasts as well as to conceal them. In 2500 BCE, warrior Minoan women on the Greek isle of Crete are depicted as wearing a bra-resembling garment that served to shove the bare breasts up and out of their clothes. The Greeks devised a bodice-type garment that tied above the breasts, leaving the breasts naked. Historical depictions of that time also show that women used a small band of material wrapped around the breasts (the apodesme) to prevent the breasts from moving; Roman women, too, apparently adopted the apodesme in their dress as well.

During the pre-Middle Ages, women were wearing a free-form, chemise-type garment that appeared to be nonconstraining. Since there was no support garment available at this time, a woman's breasts were unsupported.

By the thirteenth and fourteenth centuries, women were wearing a straight, tubular bodice, which completely flattened their breasts. This short, form-fitting bodice was worn with full skirts and full sleeves that drew the eye down and away from the breasts.

Breasts became a focal point during the Renaissance. Female attire created cleavage, and a bustline was coveted. An early version of the corset, made of whalebone and steel rods (which sounds perfectly uncomfortable), was developed. Catherine de Medici, wife of King Henry II of France, for example, is shown wearing this new device. Paintings of the time also show that a woman's breasts were tightly corseted, often with the breasts spilling out from the top of the garment. Further refinements in the corset caused the breasts to be pushed up even higher.[2]

The female breast as a sex object evolved, ironically, during the repressive Victorian era. While women were expected to cover their bodies, the style of dress was deliberately provocative. In the late nineteenth century, for example, extremely tight corsets, provocatively designed to emphasize and expose as much of the breast as possible, were the norm. The corset was an essential and constant element of female fashion. In all of its various forms, the corset actually was the dominant undergarment of support and restraint for over 350 years!

It was not until the early 1900s that a radical change in Western dress occurred with women's clothing becoming more free-form in style. To accommodate the new look, the corset gradually evolved into a more natural undergarment, which was much more comfortable to wear. Shoulder straps, rather than rigid staves, now supported the breasts. The new shoulder support, a welcome alternative to what had been available, was referred to as a brassiere. The term, brassiere, which comes from the old French word for upper arm, was first coined in 1907 by *Vogue* magazine. Before then, brassieres were known by the French term, "soutien-gorge," or "throat support" or "breast support."

In 1913, socialite Mary Phelps Jacob and her maid, Marie, devised a backless bra made from two handkerchiefs, ribbon, and cord. This lightweight, soft brassiere, albeit without cups, was the first modern-day prototype bra and was intended to flatten the breasts rather than enhance them. Her design was immediately popular with the women at the time. Years later, Ms. Jacob sold her business to Warner Brothers Corset Company for a princely sum of $1500. Perhaps she sold out too soon as Warner made over $15 million over the ensuing thirty years selling this garment.[3]

Whereas the corset accentuated the breast, the early prototype bras did not have support cups. Instead, they served to flatten the breasts, creating a look of an androgynous person. This look prevailed throughout the 1920s (flapper women generally looked flat-chested). Interestingly, during World War I, the U.S. War Industries Board requested that women stop buying corsets in order to conserve metal. This action not only helped conserve tons of metal, but it also liberated women from this tight-fitting constraint.

By the late 1920s, many companies manufactured brassieres. Bras were designed for everyday life, and the bust size categories (cup sizes) were created (one size does *not* fit all). In the 1930s and 1940s, there was a dramatic shift away from the flat-chested look to a more buxom look. The new, all-elastic bra enhanced this look by showing off a woman's curves very nicely, but it was Hollywood that created the glamorous image of full-busted movie stars. The sweater-girl look portrayed by actress Lana Turner and others, as well as the sensuous pin-up poster girl, for example, set the look and the style so popular at the time. Eyes were drawn to the breast. To enable less-endowed women to achieve a more full-figured look, falsies and the push-up bra were marketed.

Large breasts became synonymous with sex appeal, and fashion designs accentuated and exposed more of the female breast. The bullet bra created a look favored by Hollywood movie directors, and sexy imagery became Hollywood legend throughout the 1950s. But, the female liberation movement of the 1960s unleashed expressions of feminism and liberation, which, for some, included not wearing a bra. The bra-less style may have been a statement of liberation and freedom, but it certainly highlighted that part of the female anatomy—much to the delight of the opposite sex. Ironically, as the women of the time were shedding their undergarments, *Playboy* magazine and other similar male-oriented publications were showcasing female's breasts. Also, the Barbie® doll, complete with large and protruding breasts on a thin and curvaceous body, probably influenced many young girls' thoughts as to what was fashionable and desirable as well as what a female's body should look like. But attaining such a look seemed possible only from plastic surgery.

From the 1970s on, the bra was redesigned to provide comfort as well as to accent the breast. Falsies or pads could be inserted in the bra to create a more full-bodied look. It was Madonna, in the 1990s, who showed that the bra need not be hidden under clothes. She and other media stars created a new look for the bra, and many women, famous or not, followed by wearing a lacey and frilly bustier as fashion statement. The media continued to highlight full-busted women in movies, TV, and videos. Full-sized breasts were still synonymous with sex appeal.

As fashion and the media continued to focus on the female breast, many women in the 1980s and 1990s elected to have plastic surgery to enhance their appearance. Breast implants and breast augmentation surgery were embraced not only by models and movie stars but by "ordinary" women as well. For those less inclined to undergo surgery, the uplift Wonderbra helped less-endowed women create the look of someone with ample breast tissue.

The breast as a sex symbol, a symbol of eroticism, prevailed during the latter part of the twentieth century. At the same time, however, the increase in breast cancer heightened awareness that the breast is a part of the body that could become diseased. Breast cancer, benign and malignant breast disease, treatment options, and breast self-examination were openly discussed and debated. Breast health became a frequent topic of discussion among women, and breast cancer became a concern, especially among women over age fifty. In order to understand the risk factors for breast disease, including cancer, it is important to understand the structure of the breast.

## BREAST STRUCTURE

Breast tissue is composed of several elements: lobules (glandular tissue that contains cells that make and secrete milk), ducts (passageways that carry milk from the lobules to the nipple), fat (fatty tissue that surrounds the ducts and lobules), connective tissue (tough, fibrous strands that surround and support the breast), lymphatic vessels (carry clear fluid that contains immune system cells), and lymph nodes (figure 1.1). The two main types of tissues in the breast are glandular tissues and stromal (supporting) tissues. The former includes the lobules and ducts; the stromal tissue includes fatty and fibrous connective tissue. Any of these tissues can undergo changes that can result in either benign or malignant breast disease.

Breast tissue remains dormant until puberty (usually between ages nine and fourteen), when hormonal changes result in breast development. Ducts multiply and lengthen, lobules form, fat is deposited, and connective tissue increases. In short, over the course of a few short years,

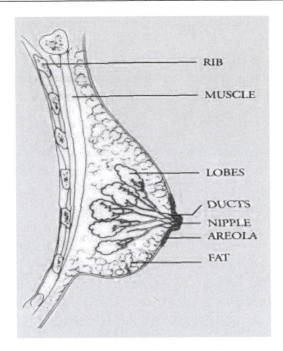

**Figure 1.1**  Diagram of the Female Breast.

the flat-chested young girl develops into a curvaceous young woman. During the reproductive years, monthly menstrual cycles cause the breasts to swell, in some cases causing discomfort and pain. During pregnancy and lactation, the breast ducts and lobules multiply. During the premenopausal years, breast tissue is generally dense. In menopause, there is a drop in hormonal stimulation, causing the glandular tissues to shrink and the breasts to become more fatty and less dense. For many women, these breast changes will pose no problems. For others, however, symptoms such as swelling and/or tenderness, breast pain, or nipple discharge may occur. Although these symptoms do not automatically mean that something is wrong, a physician should be consulted and the condition further evaluated.

## BREAST DISEASE

Most breast conditions are noncancerous and are usually characterized by a lump or an area of thickening that may or may not be palpable. Generalized breast lumpiness, sometimes described as nodular, can often be felt in the area around the nipple and areola as well as in the upper-outer part of the breast. These lumps are common, but are not life threatening per se.[4] Many premenopausal women, for example, will experience swelling, tenderness, some degree of breast discomfort or pain, or increased lumpiness as a result of extra fluid collecting in the breast tissue prior to menstruation. These symptoms usually resolve in a few days.

Some benign conditions may not cause any symptoms and may be found only during a routine physical exam or routine screening mammography. For example, some lumps are so small that they cannot be palpated but will show up on mammography or ultrasound. If the lump does not look benign, it will be labeled a suspicious lesion and further workup will be necessary. Common benign breast conditions include fibrocystic changes, fibroadenomas, and breast inflammation. Fibrocystic breast disease and fibroadenomas are the most common benign breast problems that appear as lumps.

## Fibrocystic Changes

Fibrocystic changes are the most common of benign breast conditions. Breast cysts are fluid-filled sacs caused by dilated ducts and occur most often in women between ages twenty and fifty and can be found in one or in both breasts. Large or small cysts can result when multiplying cells within breast glands and overgrowth of fibers in the supporting tissue cause a blockage in the ducts, thus preventing secretions from draining. The lump may be hard or tender, and some women may experience a sensation of fullness or a dull pain. Cysts may come and go, usually presenting before menstruation and subsiding afterward. Having one or more cysts, however, does not necessarily affect one's risk of developing breast cancer.[5] Lumpiness and tenderness fluctuate, especially among perimenopausal women, primarily because fibrocystic changes are a response to the cyclic levels of ovarian hormones.

Although the cause of fibrocystic changes is unknown, it is plausible that hormonal fluctuations in estrogen and progesterone levels contribute to the condition as many women report improvement after menopause. Some women report that their breast symptoms improve if they avoid caffeine, tea, or chocolate. Research has not confirmed that eliminating these items from one's diet has a significant impact on symptom relief, however. For those who suffer from breast swelling, some doctors recommend a reduction in salt in their diet. For those with painful cysts, drainage by fine-needle aspiration can relieve symptoms. In some cases, either a needle or surgical biopsy may be recommended to make sure that the lump is benign. Adenosis is a common finding in biopsies of women with fibrocystic changes. It refers to enlargement of breast lobules that contain more glands than usual. This condition is usually benign.

## Fibroadenomas

These benign, generally painless tumors of the breast tissues are round, firm, rubbery lumps that arise from an excess growth of glandular and connective tissues. They can be moved around easily and appear most often in adolescents and women in their twenties. This type of benign tumor can enlarge during pregnancy and breast-feeding and shrink after menopause, as they tend to respond to hormonal changes. Fibroadenomas have a typically benign appearance on mammography and can sometimes be diagnosed with fine-needle aspiration or needle core biopsy. For those tumors that grow large or change the shape of the breast, many doctors will recommend surgical removal to make sure that they are indeed benign. Since fibroadenomas can recur, it is important to have breast exams at regular intervals.

## Fat Necrosis

Fat necrosis are painless, round, and firm lumps formed by damaged and disintegrating fatty tissues. These lumps, more common in women who are obese with very large breasts, can develop in response to a bruise or blow to the breast. Fat necrosis can easily be mistaken for cancer; therefore, they should be removed by surgical biopsy.

## Sclerosing Adenosis

This benign condition frequently causes breast pain. It involves the excessive growth of tissues in the breast's lobules. Adenosis can produce lumps, which show up on mammography, often as calcifications. Because sclerosing adenosis is difficult to distinguish from cancer, the surgical biopsy is recommended.

## Nipple Discharge

Secretions or discharge from the nipple are not unusual, or even necessarily a sign of disease. Medical conditions such as thyroid dysfunction can cause a milky discharge to appear from the nipple, and oral contraceptives or other drugs, too, may cause nipple discharge. Bloody or clear discharge, however, can indicate a more serious problem that requires medical attention.

## Other Benign Breast Disease

*Mastitis* is an infection most often seen in women who are breast-feeding. The breast will feel warm, tender, and lumpy, and may appear reddish in color. The cause is usually a blocked duct that becomes inflamed and infected if not treated. Antibiotics usually cure mastitis, and warm compresses will help alleviate pain, but in some cases the duct may need to be drained.

*Epithelial hyperplasia* (proliferative breast disease) is an overgrowth of the cells that line either the ducts or the lobules. When hyperplasia involves the duct, it is referred to as ductal hyperplasia; when it involves the lobule, it is referred to as lobular hyperplasia. Hyperplasia may be grouped as usual type or atypical. Usual hyperplasia indicates a very slight increase in risk of developing breast cancer, and atypical hyperplasia occurs when cells develop in an unusual pattern. While not considered a "true" cancer, hyperplasia presents a moderate increase in risk of developing breast cancer in the future. Hyperplasia is usually found by chance, when breast tissue from a biopsy or breast surgery is examined microscopically. The overwhelming majority of biopsies performed for benign breast conditions do not contain any hyperplasia. For those who have been diagnosed with hyperplasia, it does not mean that breast cancer will necessarily develop. Regular follow-up and more frequent breast exams/mammograms would be warranted.

*Lobular carcinoma in situ (LCIS)* is not classified as breast cancer. It is a benign growth change in cells lining the lobules of the milk ducts. LCIS does not form a lump or show up on mammography; it is usually patchy throughout the breast. It is most often detected in a sample of breast tissue that has been biopsied.

Trend data from 1987 to 1999 show a rise in incidence rates of invasive lobular carcinoma, perhaps reflecting the growth in the number of women who had been taking hormone replacement therapies during this time period. The rising incidence rates of lobular breast tumors are worrisome because these tumors are more difficult to detect clinically and diagnostically. Invasive ductal carcinoma incidence rates over the same period remained essentially constant.[6] Specifically, recent data from several large-scale studies have shown that combined estrogen and progestin hormone replacement therapy is associated with a 2.0- to 3.9-fold increased risk of invasive lobular carcinoma.[7] Hormone replacement drug therapy not only increased the risk of breast cancer among postmenopausal women but also made it harder to detect. That is, it increases the risk of developing cancer while simultaneously delaying its detection. Unopposed estrogen hormone replacement, however, was not strongly associated with increased risk of LCIS.

## MALIGNANT BREAST LUMPS

There are few things more fearful than finding a lump or change in one's breast or breasts. For most women, the immediate thought is that it probably means cancer. Cancer refers to a group of diseases in which cells in the body grow, change, and multiply out of control. Thus, breast cancer is a result of erratic, uncontrolled growth and proliferation of cells that originate in the breast tissue. Breast cancer cells most likely have been growing for several years before they are large enough to be detected. If left untreated, there is a significantly greater risk of cancerous cells spreading beyond the breast to other parts of the body via the lymph system.[8] The lymphatic system plays a central role in the spread of breast cancer. The axillary (underarm) lymph nodes are particularly important as they are the first places that cancer cells are likely to be found if it has metastasized. Depending on the location of the tumor, the symptoms may include retraction of the nipple, nipple discharge, and wrinkling or dimpling of the breast skin.

Not all breast cancers are the same. Most are carcinomas, breast cancers that arise from epithelial (surface lining) tissue, and most malignant lumps develop in the mammary ducts or in the breast lobules. A very small number of breast cancers are sarcomas, which arise from the muscle, fat, or connective tissues of the breast; these are rare. Cancer of the lymphatic tissue within the breast (primary lymphoma) is also rare. Breast cancer may be noninvasive or invasive. Noninvasive breast cancer refers to cancer cells that are confined to the ducts and do not invade surrounding fatty and connective tissues of the breast. Invasive breast cancer refers to cancer cells that break through the duct and lobular wall and invade the surrounding fatty and connective tissues of the breast. It is important to note that cancer can be invasive without being metastatic. The most common form of breast cancer is ductal carcinoma in situ.

Ductal carcinoma in situ (DCIS) of the breast (also called intraductal carcinoma) is the most common type of noninvasive breast cancer. These preinvasive lesions originate within the ducts of the breast and can be detected at an early stage by screening mammography. Cancer cells that have not grown into the surrounding tissues and remain within the borders of a duct or a lobule are known as noninvasive, in situ tumors (remain in the site of origin). Generally, in situ tumors are not felt or detected because they are too tiny to have formed a lump. They are usually diagnosed by mammography. DCIS is considered a precursor to, or potential marker for, invasive ductal carcinoma.[9]

DCIS accounts for nearly 20 percent of all breast cancers detected by screening in North America.[10] Before widespread screening mammography, DCIS was diagnosed only after discovery of a palpable breast mass. Those considered most at risk for DCIS include older women (age not well defined, however), a history of benign breast disease, a family history of breast cancer, and women who do not have children or who are at an older age at the time of the first full-term pregnancy.[11] The survival rate for this cancer is extremely high. Death related to breast cancer within ten years after the diagnosis of DCIS occurs in only one to two percent of all patients.[12] Those with recurrent DCIS also have an excellent prognosis, similar to those with early stage breast cancer.[13]

Less common forms of breast cancer include *inflammatory carcinoma*, a very rare but serious and rapidly spreading type of tumor. Its symptoms, which include swelling and redness, mimic the symptoms of mastitis, a breast infection. *Paget's disease* is a rare, slow-growing cancer that begins in the ducts and spreads to the skin of the nipple and areola. This tumor may cause oozing and crustiness or itching around the nipple, but it does not involve the surrounding skin. It is typically limited to one breast. *Medullary carcinoma* (invasive breast cancer, which accounts for five percent of breast cancers), *tubular carcinoma* (special type of infiltrating carcinoma, which accounts for two percent of breast cancer diagnoses), and *mucinous carcinoma* (formed by the mucus-producing cancer cells and has a better prognosis than other breast cancers) are other forms of breast cancers.

## BREAST DISEASES ARE NOT ALIKE

Breast diseases are complex, and all cases are not the same. Unlike breast cancers, benign breast conditions are very common and are usually not life threatening. As discussed, some benign breast conditions are associated with an increased risk of developing breast cancer. Therefore, it is prudent to know one's body and to be attuned to changes in the shape, feel, or appearance of one's breasts. Any new noticeable change, thickening, or localized swelling in the breast should be brought to the physician's attention. Aside from a suspicious lump in the breast, other signs of breast disease include a spontaneous clear or bloody discharge from the nipple, retraction or indentation of the nipple, change in the size or contours of the breast, a flattening or indentation of the skin over the breast, pitting of skin over the breast (table 1.1).

At different times of the month there can be breast pain, tenderness, and swelling, but these symptoms are probably related to extra fluid that collects in the breast tissue before, during, or after the menstrual period. If, however, any one of these symptoms does not disappear before the next menstrual cycle, a physician should be consulted. There is usually no need to panic as 85 percent of all breast lumps are benign. It is the other 15 percent that need to be attended to.

**Table 1.1**
**Breast Changes and Warning Signs**

- Any new lump found in the breast or armpit.
- Any lump or thickening that does not shrink or lessen after menstruation.
- Any change in the size, shape, or symmetry of the breast(s).
- A thickening or swelling of the breast(s).
- Any dimpling, puckering, or indention in the breast(s).
- Any change in the breast skin or nipple.
- Any redness or scaliness of the nipple or breast skin.
- Any nipple discharge.
- Any nipple tenderness or pain that is different from that before or during menstruation.

## WEB SITES FOR FURTHER INFORMATION

http://Imaginis.com/breasthealth/breast
http://www.nlm.nih.gov
http://www.breastdiseases.com
http://www.breastcancer.org
http://www.cancer.org

## CHAPTER 2

# The Epidemiology of Breast Cancer: Who Is at Risk?

Forty percent of women in the United States will be diagnosed at some time in their life with a cancer (other than a superficial skin cancer), and 20 percent will die from this disease. Cancer is the second leading cause of death among men and women, second only to deaths due to heart disease. Breast cancer is the most common cancer among women in the United States and is the second most frequent cause of cancer mortality (lung cancer tops the list). This disease accounts for one-third of all cancer diagnoses and 15 percent of cancer deaths in American women.[1] In the United States, the incidence of breast cancer has been steadily increasing. From 1940 to 1982, for example, the incidence increased a modest one percent per year. However, from 1982 on, there has been an increase of four percent per year.

Many factors have contributed to the increase in breast cancer in the United States, but the recent widespread use of mammogram screening is largely responsible for detecting breast cancer at an early stage. Early detection increases the likelihood the cancer will be identified at a more treatable stage rather than at a later stage when the likelihood of spread, for example, is greater. Since mortality rates are directly related to the stage at which the cancer is detected, early diagnosis clearly affords the patient a greater chance of long-term survival. Women diagnosed and treated for breast cancer at an early stage have an excellent prognosis for long-term survival.

The American Cancer Society (ACS) as well as the National Cancer Institute's Surveillance Epidemiology and End Results (SEER) Cancer Registry, both rich sources of information, have compiled statistics from which much of the data presented in this chapter is based. Since 1963, the ACS has published its annual Cancer Facts and Figures, which is an excellent source from which to monitor long-term trends in incidence, prevalence, and mortality rates. The SEER program is an epidemiologic surveillance system, consisting of population-based tumor registries designated to track cancer incidence and survival in geographically defined areas in the United States. The registries collect information about all primary cancers.

The ACS estimates that in 2004, approximately 215,990 new cases of invasive breast cancer (all stages) were diagnosed among women in the United States. An additional 59,390 women were diagnosed with DCIS. While the overwhelming majority of breast cancer cases are diagnosed in women, the disease occurs in men as well, representing less than one percent of all cancers in males. While the rise in breast cancer among women is well documented, a new study based on SEER data from 1973 to 1998 found a disturbing and unexplainable increase in breast cancer among men. The incidence of male breast cancer rose from 0.86 per 100,000 males in 1973 to 1.08 per 100,000 males in 1998.[2] Certainly the rise in the incidence of breast cancer among women over this same time period is greater, but the increase among males is surprising. It could be that the rise in obesity among men is a contributory factor. Fat cells produce estrogen, and breast cancer in both sexes is associated with the hormone estrogen. The ACS estimates that 1,450 cases of breast cancer will be diagnosed in men in 2004 and that 470 will die from the disease in 2004.[3]

## WHAT ARE THE RISK FACTORS FOR BREAST CANCER?

A risk factor increases one's chance of getting a disease. For example, smoking is a risk factor for lung cancer. Elevated cholesterol is a risk factor for heart disease. Some risk factors cannot be changed (e.g., age, ethnicity, genetics), while other risk factors relating to personal choice can be changed (e.g., stop smoking, improve one's diet, increase one's physical activity). Epidemiology is the science that not only quantifies whether a certain disease is associated with certain risk factors, but also to what extent a risk factor increases the chances of developing a disease (the strength of association). That is, if an association between a risk factor and the development of a disease exists, how strong is that association? What are the implications for those with or without the risk factor?

Epidemiology is a population-based science that relies on data obtained from individuals but cannot specifically state with certainty that one specific individual will develop a specific disease. The focus is to identify risk factors and determinants of disease among population groups, but not among individuals per se. Determining causation and identifying risks for disease is an inexact science, and uncertainty in findings, even from the most rigorous studies, exists.

Although studies have identified several risk factors as being more compelling or significant for breast cancer, not every woman with any of these risk factors will develop the disease, and there are women with few if any breast cancer risk factors who develop the disease. Only a small portion of breast cancer cases can be explained by known risk factors. Based on probability statistics, the lifetime risk of a woman being diagnosed with breast cancer in the United States is estimated to be 12.8 percent. That is, a woman who is born today and lives to be eighty-five years of age has a 1 in 8 lifetime risk of developing breast cancer. Her lifetime risk of dying from this disease is 3.3 percent. A woman in her thirties has a 1 in 250 probability of developing breast cancer before age forty, and a woman in her sixties has a 1 in 36 probability of developing breast cancer before she reaches the age of seventy. These estimates are based on population averages, and, as such, an individual's risk may be higher or lower depending on her own personal risk factors.

Based on the available evidence from thousands of epidemiological studies focusing on breast cancer, several risk factors for this disease have been identified.

## Age

Age is an important predictor of breast cancer risk, because risk increases as one gets older. Three-quarters of women with breast cancer are over age fifty at time of diagnosis. Only 0.3 percent of breast cancer cases occur among women between ages of twenty and twenty-nine. Table 2.1 shows the odds of being diagnosed with breast cancer by age without regard for ethnic status or other risk factors.[4] When ethnicity is taken into account, the risks are different. Table 2.2 shows the estimated risk of developing breast cancer at age fifty among women of different ethnic

## Table 2.1
## The Odds of Breast Cancer Increase with Age

By age 30: 1 out of 2,212
By age 40: 1 out of 235
By age 50: 1 out of 54
By age 60: 1 out of 23
By age 70: 1 out of 14
By age 80: 1 out of 10
        Ever: 1 out of 8

*Source:* Feuer, EJ, Wun, LM. DEVCAN: Probability of
Developing or Dying of Cancer. Version 4.0. Bethesda,
MD: National Cancer Institute. 1999.

backgrounds.[5] White women age fifty have a greater risk of developing breast cancer within ten years or within twenty years compared to Hispanic, African American, or Asian women. Hispanic women at age fifty have a 1 in 63 chance of developing breast cancer within ten years compared to white women age fifty, who have a 1 in 34 chance. Therefore, it is important to understand the need to look at the data by subgroups (age or ethnicity, for example) so as not to get a mistaken impression that all women have an equal chance of developing breast cancer. All women are not created equal in this regard.

## Table 2.2
## Estimated Risk of Developing Invasive Breast Cancer
## by Age and Race

|  | Risk within 10 years | Risk within 20 years |
|---|---|---|
| Hispanic age 50 | 1 in 63 | 1 in 27 |
| Asian age 50 | 1 in 51 | 1 in 26 |
| African American age 50 | 1 in 43 | 1 in 20 |
| White age 50 | 1 in 34 | 1 in 15 |

*Source:* Morris, CR, Wright, WE, Schlag, ED. The Risk of Developing Breast Cancer Within the Next 5, 10, or 20 Years of a Woman's Life. American Journal of Preventive Medicine 20:214–18. 2001.

## Age of Menarche

Studies have shown a modest elevation in breast cancer risk associated not only with early age of menarche (age twelve or younger) but also with age when "regular" or predictable menstruation is established.[6] Among women with early menarche who had regular cycles within their first menstrual year, breast cancer risk was more than four times greater than among women with late menarche (age thirteen and older) and a long duration of irregular cycles. This finding suggests that early onset of regular ovulatory menstrual cycles, as opposed to a longer delay in the onset of regular cycles, increase a woman's risk of breast cancer.

## Age at Menopause

Breast cancer incidence rates increase more slowly after menopause. Late age at menopause is associated with greater breast cancer risk. Breast cancer risk is two times greater for those who experience menopause at age fifty-five or older than for those who experienced menopause at age forty-five or younger.[7] However, surgical menopause (removal of ovaries) markedly reduces breast cancer risk. Hysterectomy without removal of ovaries is not protective nor does it affect breast cancer risk.

## Ethnicity

It is well known that breast cancer risk, incidence, stage at diagnosis, and mortality vary considerably among ethnic groups. Table 2.3, for example, shows the stage at diagnosis of breast cancer among ethnic groups. Whereas the rate of localized breast cancer (per 100,000 women) was much higher among white women compared to African American women and Hispanic/Latina women, rates of regional and distant breast cancers (per 100,000 women) were much higher for nonwhite women compared to white women. Specifically, the rate of localized breast cancer is shown to be 90.2 per 100,000 white women compared to 65.6 per 100,000 African American women and 50.7 per 100,000 Hispanic/Latina women. However, the rate of non-localized (distant) breast cancer is shown to be 7.5 per 100,000 white women compared to 10.6 per 100,000 African American women and 6.2 per 100,000 Hispanic/Latina women. The explanations for this finding are not terribly clear.

**Table 2.3**
**Stage at Diagnosis of Breast Cancer by Race and Ethnicity, 1996–2000 (rate per 100,000)**

|  | Localized | Regional | Distant |
|---|---|---|---|
| White | 90.2 | 39.8 | 7.5 |
| African American | 65.6 | 40.6 | 10.6 |
| Hispanic/Latina | 50.7 | 29.2 | 6.2 |
| American Indian and Alaska Native | 32.4 | 19.9 | 4.8 |
| Asian American and Pacific Islander | 63.1 | 28.2 | 4.3 |

*Source*: Ries, LAG, Eisner, MP, Kosary, CL, et al. (eds). SEER Cancer Statistics Review, 1975–2000. Bethesda, MD: National Cancer Institute. http://seer.cancer.gov/csr/1975_ 2000,2003.

A large-scale research study conducted in 2004 confirmed what many in the field of medicine and epidemiology have suspected. An individual's ethnic background does indeed make a difference and is an important factor in her breast cancer diagnosis, treatment, and survival.[8] Researchers examined data collected from 1992 to 1998 on almost 125,000 women across the United States and documented significant differences in timely and appropriate treatment as well as stage of diagnosis.

The data showed that breast cancer among white women is diagnosed at an earlier, more localized stage, affording a more favorable prognosis perhaps because of early and effective of treatment or perhaps because of differences in the histology or aggressiveness of the tumor. Appropriate and timely treatment translates into better survival odds for breast cancer patients, regardless of ethnicity. While overall African American and Hispanic women tend to have breast cancer diagnosed at a later stage, the study findings also showed important differences within ethnic categories. Within the Hispanic category, for example, Puerto Rican women fared the worst, with late-stage diagnosis 3.6 times higher than the rest of the women in the Hispanic category.

Among ethnic groups, there were differences in quality of treatment received. Across the board, the African American, Hispanic, and Native American women were not only much more likely to have been diagnosed with late-stage tumors, but also to have received what was deemed to be substandard care. Puerto Rican and Mexican women were 50 percent more likely to receive substandard care when compared to non-Hispanic

white women and African American women. Perhaps access to care issues, language issues, or cultural factors might explain these results.

Asian women (Japanese, Filipino, Chinese, Korean, and Vietnamese)
had lower rates of breast cancer and were more likely to receive appropriate medical treatment compared to the other ethnic groups. But,
within this ethnic category, the Japanese women were 30 percent less
likely to be diagnosed with late-stage breast cancer, while women of
Filipino, Hawaiian, and Indian-Pakistani descent were more likely to be
diagnosed with late-stage breast cancer, especially when compared to
non-Hispanic white women. The Japanese women, for example, have
resided in the United States for longer periods of time compared to the
more recent immigrants from Asia. Recent immigrants may have less
access to care, may lack health insurance, may have a language barrier,
or may have other cultural issues that hamper their ability to seek timely
care.

There is considerable controversy as to whether differences in breast
cancer diagnosis and survival are attributable to ethnicity or to socioeconomic status (SES) or to some combination thereof. To what extent
does SES explain these differences among ethnic groups? SES is strongly
correlated with ethnicity, making it difficult to assess whether differences
are due to an individual's ethnic background solely, to the individual's
economic status solely, or to some combination thereof. There are inherent differences in an individual's lifestyle and diet, which are also
influenced by SES. To what extent these factors increase the risk of
breast cancer within specific ethnic groups needs to be considered.

One study, attempting to disentangle the influence of ethnicity and SES
on breast cancer stage, treatment, and survival, linked data from the Met-
ropolitan Detroit SEER registry to Michigan Medicaid enrollment files.[9] The
study found that before controlling for Medicaid enrollment and poverty,
African American women had a higher likelihood than white women of
unfavorable breast cancer outcomes. But, after controlling for these factors,
the African American women were not statistically significantly different
from white women on most outcomes. This implies that ethnicity, per se, was
not statistically significantly associated with unfavorable breast cancer outcomes; rather, low SES was associated with late-stage breast cancer at diagnosis, type of treatment received, and death. Poverty—regardless of one's
ethnic group—is a risk factor for breast cancer diagnosis, treatment, and
death even when other factors are taken into account.

## Genetics

Most people assume that whether they get cancer or not has something to do with their genes. Briefly, every individual inherits two copies (alleles) of every gene—one from the mother's egg and one from the father's sperm. Breast cancer is thought to arise from a series of genetic alternations (mutations) that accumulate in a cell over the course of a lifetime. Although some mutations may be inherited, most occur later in life. Depending on the particular genes and mutations involved, the breast cell may become a cancer.[10]

Familial history of breast cancer has long been suspected as being an important risk factor for the disease. Early observations of women who died of breast cancer indicated that these women were more likely than others to have had family members with breast cancer. These descriptive reports of familial aggregation of breast cancer led to empirical statistical studies that have helped understand the association between genetic risk and the development of breast cancer. Risk of breast cancer seems to be higher among women who have a first-degree relative (mother, sister, daughter) with breast cancer. Having two first-degree relatives further increases the risk.

With advances in molecular biology, the potential to identify genes that increase the risk of cancers is now possible. Several genes have been identified in inherited susceptibility to breast cancer. The two most known susceptibility genes for breast cancer are BRCA1 (breast cancer gene 1) and BRCA2 (breast cancer gene 2). A woman with a BRCA1 or BRCA2 mutation has an increased risk of developing breast cancer. Whereas the risk of breast cancer by age fifty in the general population is 2 percent, those with BRCA1 mutation have an 18 percent risk. Those with BRCA2 mutation have a six percent risk of getting breast cancer. By age eighty, the risk of breast cancer in the general population is 13.2 percent, but among women with BRCA1mutation, the risk is 59 percent. Those with a BRCA2 mutation have a 38 percent risk of breast cancer.[11] The risk for ovarian cancer, too, is elevated among BRCA1 and BRCA2 mutation carriers (table 2.4). There is an estimated 82 percent lifetime risk of breast cancer among female mutation carriers.[12]

How common are BRCA1 and BRCA2 mutations in the general population? It is estimated that 1 in 300 to 1 in 800 American women inherit a BRCA1 or BRCA2 mutation, however, certain mutations in

**Table 2.4**
**Risk of Breast Cancer Among BRCA1 and BRCA2 Carriers**

|  | BRCA1 | BRCA2 | General Population |
|---|---|---|---|
| Risk of breast cancer by age 50 | 18% | 6% | 2% |
| Risk of breast cancer by age 80 | 59% | 38% | 13.2% |
| Risk of ovarian cancer by age 50 | 12% | 3% | 0.3% |
| Risk of ovarian cancer by age 80 | 58% | 36% | 1.7% |

*Source:* Scheuer, L, Kauff, N, Robson, M, et al. Outcome of Preventive Surgery and Screening for Breast and Ovarian Cancer in BRCA Mutation Carriers. Journal of Clinical Oncology, Mar 1:1260–68. 2002.

these genes have been identified more frequently in specific population groups.[13] In particular, Ashkenazi Jewish women appear to be at greater risk of inheriting these mutations than other ethnic groups. These women appear to be at higher risk regardless of family history or lifestyle. A study that conducted a molecular analysis on a sample of Ashkenazi Jewish women with inherited BRCA1 and BRCA2 mutations calculated the lifetime risk of breast cancer among female mutation carriers in this sample to be 82 percent. Breast cancer risk by age fifty among mutation carriers in this sample who were born before 1940 was 24 percent, but among those born after 1940, the risk increased to 67 percent.[14] Explanations for this finding are not clear.

It must be stressed that most breast cancer occurs in the absence of a BRCA1 or BRCA2 mutation. Although inheritance of a BRCA1 or BRCA2 mutation is an important contributor to breast cancer, this does not necessarily mean that a woman will develop this disease. She is at increased *risk* of developing the disease. The genetic factors that influence disease development among women who inherit a BRCA1 or BRCA2 susceptibility allele are not yet known, but research on potential mechanisms that could explain how the genes interact to increase the risk of breast or ovarian cancer is being conducted. Of course other factors may influence the development of breast cancer, and, if these factors could be modified, then the risk of breast cancer among women inheriting a susceptibility allele could be reduced. For example, use of oral contraceptives has been associated with an increased risk of breast cancer among women with susceptibility alleles. Therefore, stopping the use of oral contraceptives could modify BRCA1- and BRCA2-related breast cancer risk.

Other susceptibility genes have been associated with increased risk of breast cancer. Inherited mutations in the p53 tumor suppressor gene have been associated with an increased risk of developing breast cancer. The p53 mutations can also increase the risk of developing other cancers such as leukemia, brain tumors, and cancer of bones or connective tissue. Another gene, ATM (ataxia-telangiectasia mutation), might also lead to inherited breast cancer. More studies must be conducted in order to clarify the role of these genetic mutations in the development of breast cancer. As more becomes known about genetic changes and the development of breast cancer, more targeted treatments and preventive measures will emerge.

Many people hesitate to undergo genetic testing, and many physicians hesitate to offer it primarily because of insurance concerns. If genetic testing discovers a cancer risk, for example, that information could be used against an individual when obtaining health insurance coverage. However, with genetic information, an individual at high risk could better decide whether or not to elect preventive care, to take protective action. There is a trade-off between knowing "too much" and not knowing.

## Breasts and Benign Breast Disease

Evidence suggests a relationship between breast tissue characteristics in individual women and increased risk of breast cancer. On mammogram, the breast is defined by the visualized relative amounts of fat, connective tissue, and epithelial tissue. Fat appears as radiologically lucent areas, whereas connective and epithelial tissue appear as areas of high radiologic density. Women with denser breasts (containing more connective and glandular tissue) are at higher risk for breast cancer; women with breasts that are less dense (contain more fatty tissue) appear not to be, perhaps because less dense breasts are easier to assess with mammography. A poorly differentiated breast cancer tumor that is 1 cm in diameter is easily diagnosed in a breast containing substantial fat tissue (not dense), but this same tumor would be difficult to detect in a dense breast. But, there are clearly other risk factors that could account for elevated risk. The absolute increase in risk of breast cancer for women with dense breasts is small.[15]

Having a previous breast biopsy result of atypical hyperplasia (cells that develop in an unusual pattern) increases the risk of breast cancer four to five times. Those whose biopsies detected proliferative breast disease (group of noncancerous conditions that may increase the risk of developing breast cancer; e.g., ductal hyperplasia, lobular hyperplasia) without atypical or usual hyperplasia (increased growth in the size and number of normal cells within either the ducts or lobes) have a slightly elevated risk of breast cancer (1.5 to 2 times greater than other women). However, fibrocystic changes in the breast without proliferative breast disease do not affect one's breast cancer risk.[16]

Do breast implants increase the risk of breast cancer? The consensus is that there appears that there is no elevated cancer risk among those with silicone breast implants; but, implants do make it harder to see breast tissue on standard mammograms.

## Breast-Feeding

Breast-feeding has been thought to be a protective factor in the development of breast cancer. Breast-feeding may cause hormonal changes, particularly a decrease in the level of estrogen. As such, a woman's risk of developing breast cancer may be reduced as a result of lower estrogen levels. Breast-feeding also suppresses ovulation, which could affect the number of ovulatory cycles a woman would have over the course of her reproductive life. Women who have fewer ovulatory cycles may have a decreased risk of developing breast cancer.

Breast-feeding may cause physical changes in the cells that line the mammary ducts, which may make the cells more resistant to mutations that could lead to cancer. However, it is difficult to say with certainty whether it is the breast-feeding that confers protection or a combination of other factors. Study results vary primarily because of study design and study population differences. Some studies have shown that breast-feeding was more protective against the development of breast cancer among premenopausal women as compared to postmenopausal women, while others showed no overall reduction in breast cancer risk associated with breast-feeding. The risk of premenopausal breast cancer among women forty years of age or younger was nearly 35 percent lower among those who breast-fed for more than fifteen months compared to those who did not breast-feed their children. Postmenopausal women who had breast-fed for more than fifteen months had a 30 percent lower risk of breast cancer than postmenopausal women who never breast-fed.[17] It is not clear why breast-feeding should be more protective against premenopausal breast cancer than postmenopausal breast cancer. At this time, the literature is inconclusive as to the benefits breast-feeding confers on breast cancer development.

## Obesity, Diet, and Physical Activity

Research shows that there is a direct relationship between excess weight and risk of death from most cancers. In 2003, a sixteen-year (1982–1998) study of 900,000 initially healthy men and women was published by the ACS. The study found an association between excess body weight and many cancers including breast, colon and rectum, esophagus, pancreas, kidney, gallbladder, ovary, cervix, liver, prostate, multiple myeloma and non-Hodgkin's lymphoma.[18] Focusing specifically on breast cancer, the risk of death is 34 percent higher in a woman with a body mass index (BMI; a measure of weight in relation to height) of 25–30; 63 percent higher in a woman with a BMI of 30–35, and 70 percent higher in those with a BMI of 35–40. Being overweight apparently is associated with an increased risk of developing breast cancer, especially for postmenopausal women. Women who gained significant weight over the decades have almost twice the risk of breast cancer compared to women who had not gained weight. The risk does not seem to be as great for those who have been overweight since childhood. When smoking status was taken into account, cancer risk associated with excess weight among those who never smoked was still high.

Several studies have looked at the role of specific dietary factors in breast cancer causation (fat, fiber, antioxidants, alcohol, and caffeine intake). The data do not support the hypothesis that diet has a direct effect on breast cancer risk.[19] However, the findings do suggest that limiting alcohol consumption to two or fewer glasses of wine a day, reducing high caffeine intake, and avoiding weight gain during adult years would be beneficial.

The relationship between diet and breast cancer is complex and the results conflicting. In those countries where the diet is low in total fat, low in polyunsaturated fat, and low in saturated fat, breast cancer is less common. Conversely, high-fat diets, particularly those rich in red meats, have been linked to higher risk of cancer. The fats in fish as well as mono-unsaturated oils (olive and canola), high-fiber foods, and legumes are somewhat protective against cancer. It has been suggested that foods with high phytoestrogen content (soy products) can reduce breast cancer risk, but more research needs to be conducted to understand more fully if there is a protective effect of such a diet.

Does physical activity have a protective effect against breast cancer? Physical activity may decrease exposure of breast tissue to estrogen, a major contributor to the development of breast cancer, and it certainly would help keep the pounds off. Data from the 2000 National Health Interview Survey show that more women than men are inactive. Almost three-quarters of women do not engage in regular leisure-time physical activity, compared to two-thirds of men.[20] Research has shown that women who are physically active and engage in regular exercise have a decreased risk for breast cancer.[21] What, however, defines "physically active" or "regular exercise"? What kinds of physical activity would confer benefits? How much exercise is needed to have a protective effect? Several large-scale studies have looked at the affect exercise has on breast cancer risk and have helped clarify the issue.

Findings from the large-scale Women's Health Initiative (WHI) study (from 1993–1998) have shed light on the potential benefits of exercise on a cohort of 74,171 women aged fifty to seventy-nine years. Compared with less active women, women who engaged in 1.25 to 2.5 hours a week of brisk walking had an 18 percent decreased risk of breast cancer. A slightly greater reduction in risk was seen for women who engaged in the equivalent of ten hours or more per week of brisk walking. The data suggest that increased physical activity (even brisk walking) was associated with a reduced risk of breast cancer in postmenopausal women. Those who exercised for longer periods of time and engaged in more strenuous activity showed the most benefit. Also, women who had been physically active at ages thirty-five to fifty also experienced a reduced cancer risk.[22]

Findings from the WHI study, and other studies that also have researched the issue, show that exercise need not be vigorous in order to confer a health benefit. Whether one spends hours in the fitness club doing aerobic exercises or takes several brisk walks a week, there is a positive potential benefit to the activity. Clearly, the degree of protection is directly related to the amount of physical activity. Exercising daily or at least a few times a week not only can help reduce the risk of breast cancer, but it also can result in weight loss and significant improvements in cardiovascular fitness.

## Geographic Variation and Migrant Studies

International rates of breast cancer clearly show differences among countries. Rates are generally lowest in Asia and Africa, and highest in Western Europe, Canada, and the United States. Within the United States, there are variations in rates. Breast cancer rates are lower in the South, but recent mortality rates have increased in many areas of this region, perhaps reflecting a change in sociodemographics or environmental factors. The highest breast cancer incidence rates are in the San Francisco Bay area, suburban Chicago, and the Northeast, especially in the urban centers. Within the Northeast, Long Island, New York, had been perceived as having the highest rate of breast cancer.

In the early 1990s, Long Island women lobbied Congress successfully to fund a large population-based case-control study to identify environmental and other potential risk factors thought to contribute to the development of breast cancer in this area. Specifically, the Long Island Breast Cancer Study Project was conducted to determine whether breast cancer risk among women in the counties of Nassau and Suffolk, New York, was elevated as a result of environmental exposures.[23] This carefully designed, federally mandated study did not find statistically significant differences in risk of breast cancer for environmental toxins, but did affirm the increased risk for breast cancer for established risk factors such as family history of breast cancer (see "Environmental Exposures" section for further detail).

Migrant studies, which seek to understand the effects that lifestyle, diet, environmental, and genetic factors have on disease, have provided interesting findings on breast cancer risk. Breast cancer incidence and death rates among migrant populations appear to increase substantially after arrival in the United States. That is, over time, the risk of breast cancer among migrants approaches that among the native-born population. Since age is a known risk factor for breast cancer, it is important to take into account the age at which the individual migrated to the United States. Did migration take place before or after key reproductive-related events associated with increased risk of breast cancer (age of menarche, age at giving birth, age of menopause)? Migrants who were older when they came to the United States tend to have a lower risk than migrants who came to this country at a younger age. Further, recent migrants tend to have lower risk than migrants who have lived in the United States for twenty years or more.

## Environmental Exposures

It had been believed that certain chemicals in the environment contributed to the development of breast cancer. Probably the most comprehensive study to assess environmental factors as potential risks for breast cancer is the Long Island Breast Cancer Study Project, discussed earlier. This study was conducted to determine among other things, whether the risk of breast cancer among women living on Long Island was associated with polycyclic aromatic hydrocarbons and orgnochlorine compounds such as DDT and polychlorinated biphenyls (PCBs). In this study, blood levels of organochlorines such as PCBs or DDT were quantified. Environmental samples of water and soil were tested for chlorinated and carbamate pesticides and metals. After careful analysis, the findings did not show a clear link between breast cancer risk and exposure to environmental pollutants.[24] In fact, long-term residents (fifteen or more years living in residence) with environmental home samples did not differ from other long-term residents in the development of breast cancer.

## Oral Contraceptive Use

Because hormonal factors are known to influence the development of breast cancer and because oral contraceptives (OCs) work by manipulating hormones, there has been concern that taking OCs could increase the risk of breast cancer among women. Over 80 percent of U.S. women born since 1945 have used some type of OC at some point in their life. These women are now reaching the ages of greatest breast cancer risk. As such, it is important to assess whether there is elevated risk of breast cancer among former or current OC users.

Many epidemiological studies have investigated whether hormonal contraceptives affect breast cancer risk. The Collaborative Group on Hormonal Factors in Breast Cancer was established in 1992 to reanalyze worldwide data based on fifty-four epidemiological studies that had been conducted in twenty-five countries.[25] The study population consisted of over 53,000 women with breast cancer and over 100,000 women without breast cancer. The results provided strong evidence for two main conclusions: (1) there was a small increase in the risk of developing breast cancer among women who were taking combined OCs or had used them in the past ten years, and (2) there is no significant excess risk of developing breast cancer ten or more years after stopping OC use. Cancers diagnosed in women who had used combined OCs were less clinically advanced than those diagnosed in women who had never used OCs.

Findings from the National Institute of Child Health and Human Development Women's Contraceptive and Reproductive Experiences Study, based on data collected on over 9,000 women who were between thirty-five and sixty-four years of age, also found that women who took OCs at some point in their lives were no more likely to develop breast cancer than were women who did not. There was no increase in breast cancer risk among former and current users of OCs. Further, there was no elevated risk among ethnic groups. Age of initiation of OCs, length of time using OCs, time since last use, and use by estrogen dose also did not increase the risk of breast cancer development.[26]

## Hormones and Hormone Replacement Therapy

Hormones play a major role in the etiology of breast cancer. Estrogen, in particular, is essential for the normal growth and development of the breast. The main forms of estrogen in females (endogenous estrogen) include estradiol, the main estrogen made by the ovaries before menopause; estrone, a weaker estrogen produced both in the ovaries and in fat tissue from other hormones and is the main estrogen found in women after menopause (although the ovaries continue to produce small amounts of estradiol); and estriol, produced almost exclusively during pregnancy.

Both normal breast tissue and breast malignancies are dependent on estrogen for their growth. During each menstrual cycle, estrogen and other ovarian hormones signal cells in the breast and uterus to divide and multiply. Cumulative exposure of the breast to estrogen affects the rate of cell division. Since estrogen stimulates cell division, it can increase the chance of making a normal cell into a cancer cell. One- to two-thirds of all breast tumors has estrogen receptors and depends on estrogen for growth. Antiestrogens (such as tamoxifen), for example, can help block the binding of estrogen to its receptor and prevent that hormone from delivering its message to the breast tumor cells to divide and multiply.

The effect of estrogen on breast cancer risk was shown over one hundred years ago when researchers found that removing the ovaries of women with breast cancer improved their chances of survival. Women who have had their ovaries removed early in life have a very low incidence of breast cancer. Hence, it is hypothesized that life-long exposure to estrogen plays an important role in affecting breast cancer risk; i.e., the length of exposure to estrogen during a woman's lifetime has an effect on the development of breast cancer.

Doctors touted the use of estrogen replacement therapy (ERT; use of estrogen alone) and combined hormone replacement therapy (CHRT; estrogen plus progestin) to relieve the symptoms of menopause as the best way for older women also to protect their bones and prevent heart disease. Since the 1960s, millions of prescriptions were written for women seeking to replace the body's lost estrogen. ERT was widely used in the 1960s, but fell out of favor in the 1970s after reports showed an increase in uterine cancer among women taking this estrogen replacement. With the introduction of CHRT in the 1980s, which did not confer a risk of uterine cancer, this type of hormone replacement was widely prescribed.

While ERT and CHRT helped alleviate menopausal symptoms, its long-term risks and benefits needed to be assessed. Initially, the early observational studies, conducted in the 1980s and 1990s, highlighted the benefits of CHRT and ERT, including relief from menopausal symptoms and bone and heart protection. But mounting evidence from further study began to uncover a number of serious risks associated with taking ERT and CHRT including higher risk of heart attack, stroke, thromboembolic disorders, and cardiovascular events. Among women who took ERT, their risk of developing endometrial cancer, blood clots, stroke, and coronary disease was statistically greater than for women who did not take estrogen.[27] When progestin was added to the estrogen, the risk of endometrial cancer decreased, but the other risks persisted. Specifically, a pooled analysis of fifty-one observational studies found that current users of CHRT or progestin alone for five years or longer had a 53 percent increase in risk of breast cancer.[28] It could be that progestin added to HRT might actually increase breast cancer risk.

Observational studies are not randomized trials. What was needed was a large-scale clinical trial that would randomly assign women to treatment or to placebo groups to quantify the potential benefits and risks of CHRT and ERT. More valid comparisons could be made between outcomes among those who took CHRT or ERT and those who did not in a randomized trial. Observational studies cannot produce such evidence by virtue of their study design. The federal government agreed to fund a large-scale, multicenter trial to assess the risks and benefits of CHRT and ERT.

The Womens' Health Initiative (WHI), begun in 1993, was designed to be a fifteen-year multimillion-dollar initiative to focus on strategies for preventing heart disease, breast and colorectal cancer, and osteoporosis in postmenopausal women. The trial involved over 161,000 women between the ages of fifty and seventy-nine and had three components: (1) a randomized clinical trial that enrolled over 68,000 postmenopausal women to study the effect of hormonal therapy on the prevention of heart disease and osteoporosis and any associated risk for breast cancer. Women in this trial either took hormone pills or a placebo; (2) an observational study that would look at lifestyle, health, and risk factors and specific disease outcomes of 100,000 women; (3) a community prevention study, which consisted of approaches to developing healthful behaviors and will not be discussed here. The postmenopausal hormone therapy clinical trials had two studies: the estrogen plus progestin study of women with a uterus, and the estrogen alone study of women without a uterus. In both of these trials, women were randomly assigned to either the hormone medication being studied or to placebo. The trial was to continue for several years in order to order to assess risks and benefits on the study outcomes.

Much to the surprise of the researchers and study sponsors, the WHI trial had to be stopped because of increased risk of invasive breast cancer, stroke, and heart disease among the sample of healthy women. The findings from the WHI were so statistically compelling that the trial was halted before its intended end date because the harmful effects of CHRT exceeded the preventive benefits; women were strongly advised to discontinue HRT.[29] In brief, after 5.6 years of follow-up, the CHRT trial was terminated because of statistically significant results. In this study, 16,608 postmenopausal women were randomly assigned to CHRT or to placebo. Findings showed that the CHRT group was at greater risk of heart disease, breast cancer, stroke, and blood clots compared to the women receiving the placebo. While there were positive benefits on hip fracture and colorectal cancer, these benefits were overshadowed by the serious risks of continuing to take CHRT. The federal government advised physicians to stop prescribing CHRT.

Additional data provided by the WHI randomized trial further show that not only did combined estrogen plus progestin use increase incident of breast cancers, but these tumors were diagnosed at a more advanced stage compared with placebo use. The findings suggest that estrogen plus progestin may stimulate breast cancer growth and density of breast tissue, thus making breast cancer diagnosis more difficult and increasing the possibility that the cancer would be diagnosed at a more advanced stage, a terrible combination of increasing the risk of disease while also delaying its detection. Findings also showed a sharp increase in mammographic abnormalities among women in the estrogen plus progestin group.[30] The increased risk of breast cancer among postmenopausal women who used a combination of estrogen plus progestin hormone therapy as well as the increase in the number of mammographic abnormalities provides compelling evidence against the use of CHRT.[31] The relatively early development of more breast cancers in the CHRT group was unexpected because the observational studies suggested that breast cancer risk would increase with longer-term (greater than five years) hormonal use. The clinical trial clearly showed otherwise.

In addition to the CHRT trial, the WHI also studied the effect of estrogen-only treatment on a sample of 11,000 healthy postmenopausal women who had had a hysterectomy. This part of the WHI assessed the effect of long-term use of estrogen-only on heart disease, fractures, breast and colorectal cancer, and dementia as well. This was a randomized clinical trial, and it too was stopped after an average of seven years of follow-up because estrogen alone did not appear to protect against heart disease, a key question of the study. Estrogen-only appeared to increase the risk of stroke and there was a trend toward increased risk of dementia and/ or mild cognitive impairment. Estrogen-only apparently did not increase the risk of breast cancer during the period of study. The increased risk of stroke among healthy women was reason enough to stop the trial.[32]

Recent research findings also showed that use of combined estrogen and progestin HRT not only increases breast cancer risk, but that its use is also more strongly associated with the risk of invasive lobular breast carcinoma than that of invasive ductal carcinoma. This suggests that invasive lobular carcinoma may be more hormonally responsive than invasive ductal carcinoma.[33] The increases were most pronounced among women fifty years of age and older. This finding presents a challenge to physicians because lobular carcinoma, while less common than ductal carcinoma, is more difficult to detect. Clearly, early detection is a key component to early treatment and to increased survival.

## Tumor Size

While the above listed potential risk factors for breast cancer are generally well known, a 2003 study report prepared by the ACS unexpectedly found that the proportion of women with newly diagnosed breast cancer in the 1990s had unusually large tumors (tumors larger than 5 cm).[34] Large tumors are more likely to spread and to be fatal, hence the alarm and concern. Surprisingly, the incidence of large tumors increased by more than 2 percent a year between 1992 and 2000, but only in white women. The reason for this finding is not clear, especially since tumors in white women are generally small and localized. African American women generally tend to present at a later stage with larger tumors and generally have a poorer prognosis. Large tumors generally are approximately twice as common in African American women but the incidence of large tumors among this ethnic group did not change during the 1990s.

What could be responsible for this surprising finding? Perhaps obesity and use of HRT contributed to the growth of large cancers in white women. White women were more likely to take HRT compared to African American women. But, African American women tend to be overweight, which would put them at risk.

## Diethylstilbestrol (DES)

Use of DES by pregnant women, particularly in the 1940s and 1950s, and its relationship to the development of breast cancer in their daughters has been studied. A cohort of DES daughters was studied because it was thought that they would be at greater risk of developing breast cancer compared to women whose mothers did not take DES. While not definitive, study findings show that being exposed to DES before birth may be associated with an increased risk of breast cancer. Although there was a higher incidence of breast cancer among those exposed to DES, the results were not statistically significant, implying that chance rather than exposure is an explanation. The prospective follow-up study found that DES daughters under age forty did not have a higher risk of breast cancer, while DES daughters over age forty were 2.5 times more likely to have breast cancer than unexposed women over forty. Caution in interpreting the findings is warranted because the median age of the study group was forty-three years; the cohort has not yet reached the prime ages when breast cancer can develop.[35]

## Alcohol Use

Studies have suggested a weak yet positive association between alcohol consumption and breast cancer risk. Compared with nondrinkers, women who drink one alcoholic drink a day have a small increase in risk, while those who have two to five drinks a day have 1.5 times the risk of women who drink no alcohol. It seems that no specific type of alcoholic drink was more predictive of increased risk than any other. There might be confounding factors that would explain this relationship, however.[36]

## Smoking

Although tobacco has been shown to elevate the risk of many cancers, there appears not to be any association with breast cancer risk.

## BREAST CANCER MORTALITY

A diagnosis of cancer is not an automatic death sentence by any stretch of the imagination. As a result of advances in treatment and therapeutics, many cancers have a very favorable prognosis as is best typified by cancer-specific survival rates. There is good news to report on breast cancer mortality in the United States. Although breast cancer incidence rates continue to increase among women of all ethnic backgrounds, overall breast cancer mortality has been steadily decreasing, especially since 1989. Breast cancer death rates peaked in the late 1980s and then decreased on average by 1.4 percent per year in the early 1990s and more rapidly (by 3.2 percent per year) from 1995 to 1999.[37] The explanation for this trend in breast cancer death rates is not well understood, but may be a result of early detection and treatment.

Breast cancer mortality rates, not surprisingly, vary by age. In the 1990s, rates significantly decreased across all ages, except for women younger than age thirty, who experienced nonsignificant declines, and for women age eighty-five and older, who had level rates. From 1987 to 1997, annual breast cancer death rate per 100,000 women younger than age fifty decreased 19 percent while for women aged fifty to sixty-nine, the decrease was 18 percent. Among older women aged seventy and seventy-nine, the decrease was 9 percent. The sharp decrease since 1987 is most probably due to the changes in breast cancer diagnostic and treatment methods.[38]

ACS trend data from the 1950s to 1975 show that, while breast cancer mortality rates among white women remained relatively constant, rates among nonwhite women increased steadily. From 1975 to 2000, breast cancer mortality among white women decreased from 31.8 percent to 26.3 percent, while the African American rate increased from 29.5 percent to 34.6 percent. Further research is needed to understand more fully the disparity in breast mortality rates and why they differ so significantly among ethnic groups. A combination of factors is likely to contribute to the differences, but the bottom line is that one's ethnicity is a predictor of adverse breast cancer outcome.

Differences in mammography use may contribute to ethnic differences in breast cancer mortality. Whereas the percentage of women age forty and over having a mammogram within the past two years (2002 baseline) was 70.3 percent, there are differences among ethnic groups: 72.1 percent of white women and older had a mammogram within the past two years compared to 67.9 percent of African American women and 61.4 percent of Hispanic women. When SES was taken into account, only 55.2 percent of women forty and over who were below the federal poverty level had a mammogram within the past two years, compared to 72.2 percent of women forty and over who were at or above the federal poverty level.[39] Many factors such as lack of health insurance, low education level, and low health literacy could explain these findings.

## SURVIVAL RATES

Although the number of new cases of breast cancer (incident cases) continues to increase, many more women are breast cancer survivors (prevalent cases), and much of the success in prolonging life after a diagnosis of breast cancer can be attributed to early detection and treatment. Certainly, surgery followed by radiation and/or chemotherapy has contributed to increased survival, and the use of tamoxifen and other drugs that block hormones from nurturing the cancer have been found to increase survival and to cut the risk of relapse significantly.

Declining breast cancer mortality rates have been observed in the United States as well as in other developed nations. What this means is that there are many more women today surviving breast cancer than was the case a decade ago. Survival is conventionally delineated by five-year survival rates. That is, a five-year survival rate refers to the average number of individuals who are still alive five years after diagnosis. It is important to stress that survival rates are based on averages, and some women will live longer than others. Logically, survival depends on many factors including the type of breast cancer, the size and location of the cancer, whether the cancer was diagnosed at an early or more advanced stage, and individual risk factors.

SEER and the ACS data show that survival rates have improved for virtually all age and ethnic groups. The ACS estimates that the five-year survival rate among women younger than age forty-five is 81 percent, and among those between the ages of forty-five and sixty-four, the five-year survival rate is 85 percent. Among those women age sixty-five and older, the five-year survival rate is 86 percent. Younger women tend to have more aggressive breast cancers, which may explain why their survival rates are lower than that for older women. Women, regardless of age, who are diagnosed with early-stage breast cancer have close to a 100 percent five-year survival rate, while those with more advanced breast cancer have poorer survival rates.

It has long been thought that one's ethnic background can have a direct effect on survival. Findings from one of the largest and most comprehensive studies to evaluate the relationship between ethnicity/race and breast cancer stage, treatment, and survival clearly showed that African Americans, Hispanics, and Native Americans had poorer survival rates compared to non-Hispanic white women and Asian women. The African American and Hispanic women had a 10 to 70 percent greater risk of dying after a breast cancer diagnosis compared to non-Hispanic whites.[40] Even though this disparity has been noted for many years, the trend persists and remains an important problem. Perhaps rather than biological factors, socioeconomic factors and access to care issues explain this disparity.

## SUMMARY

Each year over 200,000 women in the United States are diagnosed with breast cancer. This represents approximately one-third of all cancers diagnosed in American women. Although the mechanisms of breast cancer development are not understood fully, many variables such as age, ethnicity, heredity, diet, culture, and SES have been shown to be risk factors for the disease. While the overall breast cancer survival rate has increased substantially over the years, there are variations among ethnic groups. Overall, breast cancer is detected earlier and at a less advanced stage in white women as compared to African American and Hispanic women. Early diagnosis and treatment confer benefits; those women who are diagnosed with localized cancer have a much higher survival rate than those who present with more advanced cancer.

Many risk factors can influence a woman's risk of developing breast cancer. In particular, women over age fifty are at greatest risk as are women of any age whose mother or sister has had breast cancer, particularly if the cancer occurred when the patient was premenopausal. Women with precancerous breast disease are at higher risk of breast cancer, too. But, having one or more of these risk factors does not necessarily mean that a woman is destined to develop breast cancer. In fact, the majority of women with breast cancer have none of the apparent risk factors, and many women who do have known risk factors are cancer free. Risk is based on probability and population averages. It does not imply inevitability. Furthermore, advances in cancer detection as well as exciting advances in treatment have enabled many cancer survivors to live many years with an excellent quality of life.

## WEB SITES FOR FURTHER INFORMATION

http://www.seer.cancer.org
http://www.acs.org
http://www.nlm.nih.gov

## CHAPTER 3

# Breast Cancer and Treatment Options

Few diseases evoke as much fear as does breast cancer. Many women perceive the diagnosis of breast cancer as a death sentence despite the remarkable strides made in breast cancer detection and treatment and breast cancer survival. In the United States, more women seem to be afraid of developing breast cancer than of having a heart attack. Yes, the diagnosis of breast cancer can be devastating, but this disease is not uniformly fatal, and there are some very effective treatment options. The type of treatment naturally will be dictated by many factors including patient characteristics, disease characteristics, and hormone receptor status. This chapter provides an overview of breast cancer treatment options based on the most current information available. Medical research is making great strides in unlocking the secrets of breast cancer with new techniques for diagnosis, new treatment modalities, and advances in molecular genetics providing answers to as yet unanswered questions. But, with new information published each month, some of the material presented that is considered cutting-edge today may be out of date one year from now.

## CANCER STAGING

Breast cancer cases are not all the same. Staging of a cancer, the process used to assess the size, location, and pattern of cancer, is an important indicator of the extent of cancer growth and is often crucial for identifying appropriate treatment options. It also helps physicians discern prognosis. Although staging of a cancer is important, prognosis and treatment options often are influenced by other factors such as age and comorbid conditions. Not every woman with the same staging receives the same treatment or has the same prognosis. Findings from imaging studies, results of the surgical biopsy, and material included in the pathology report help determine the severity of a cancer.

The following presents a very brief description of overall staging categories and subcategories.[1]

1. Stage 0, or in situ, meaning in place, represents very early breast cancer, which has not spread beyond the breast ductal system. One type of Stage 0 cancer is ductal carcinoma in situ (DCIS). The overall relative five-year survival rate for Stage 0 cancer is 100 percent.

2. Stage I refers to the original cancer that is no larger than 2 cm in size and has not spread outside of the breast tissue to the lymph nodes. Stage I is considered early breast cancer with an overall relative five-year survival rate of 98 percent.

3. Stage IIA refers to a cancerous tumor between 2 and 5 cm in diameter that has not spread to the lymph nodes. Stage IIB refers to a tumor that is between 2 and 5 cm in diameter that has spread to the axillary lymph nodes. The relative five-year survival rate for Stage IIA is 88 percent and for Stage IIB, 76 percent.

4. Stage IIIA and IIIB refer to a cancer that is smaller than 5 cm and has spread to the lymph nodes under the arm as well as spreading to other lymph nodes, or the cancer is larger than 5 cm and has spread to the lymph nodes under the arm. In Stage IIIB, the cancer that has spread to tissues near the breast (skin, chest wall, for example), or the cancer has spread to lymph nodes inside the chest wall along the breast bone. For Stage IIIA cancers, the relative five-year survival rate is 56 percent and 49 percent for Stage IIIB.

5. Stage IV, the most serious staging, refers to a cancer that has spread to other parts of the body (bone, lung, liver, brain), or the tumor has spread locally to the skin and lymph nodes inside the neck near the collarbone. Relative five-year survival for Stage IV breast cancer is 16 percent.

Other factors, too, are taken into account in the staging process; that is, the tumor size, the number of palpable nodes, and any metastasis.

A specific system to stage breast cancer relies on the T/N/M system. "T" refers to the size of the tumor and whether or not it is well contained or has spread to surrounding tissues. "N" refers to lymph node involvement; whether or not the tumor has spread into the surrounding lymph nodes, the number of nodes involved, and their size. "M" refers to the extent of distant metastases. For example, a T1, N0, M0 tumor refers to a tumor that is 2 cm or less in diameter, there is no spread to the lymph nodes, there are no distant metastasis to other organs. Such a classification would most likely be labeled as a stage I cancer, which has a very good prognosis. This system, too, gives an indication of prognosis and helps physicians make treatment decisions.

## TREATMENT OPTIONS

Once a breast lump is detected and diagnosed, most women have a number of treatment options available. Each option has its advantages and disadvantages, and each has side effects. Because of the different stages of breast cancer and different types of cancer, there is not one specific treatment that is best for all breast cancer patients. Often different types of treatment are used in combination simultaneously or sequentially. Which treatment or treatments are recommended will depend on a number of factors including the tumor size and histologic type, lymph node status, biomarkers (measurable parameters in tissues, cells, or fluids), stage of disease, hormone receptor status, and personal characteristics of the individual including age, menopausal status, risk for breast cancer, and health status.

While the clinical parameters of the disease usually dictate the type of treatment option, an individual's input about treatment options is very important. Individual patients differ in the importance they place on the risks and benefits of treatment. Self-image, lifestyle, and quality of life needs are important considerations that must be taken into account. As such, treatment decisions must be made with an individual patient's input in concert with her doctor's guidance.

Whatever the treatment option, be it surgery, radiation, chemotherapy and/or hormonal treatment, the goal is the same: to kill the cancer cells. Surgery and radiation are local treatments as they are directed at one area of the breast, whereas chemotherapy and hormonal therapy are systemic treatments as they target the entire body. The treatments may be given individually or in some combination, either simultaneously or sequentially, depending on a host of factors.

## Surgical Treatment

Surgery is often the first line of treatment for many of the solid tumors. In some cases, surgical excision may be sufficient without other forms of treatment. In other instances, surgical resection is usually followed by a course of radiation and/or chemotherapy. There are different surgical options available depending on the nature and type of the cancerous growth.

Sentinel node lymphoscintigraphy is an important method to determine if any of the axillary lymph nodes (under the armpit) contain cancerous cells. Since the axillary lymph nodes are the primary drainage sites for the breast, once a diagnosis of breast cancer is made, most patients with invasive breast cancer most probably will undergo axillary biopsy and possible dissection. While this procedure provides important information about the staging of the cancer, it can produce side effects, notably arm swelling and possible infections. Sentinel node lymphoscintigraphy is a technique to identify the sentinel node or nodes in the axillary lymph system. The sentinel node concept is based on the premise that a breast tumor drains into one or two key, or sentinel, lymph nodes before drainage continues to the other lymph nodes. Injecting a radioactive dye and a blue colorant (to help in visualization), the radiologist and surgeon can identify the sentinel node or nodes, which are surgically removed and tested for cancer cells. If the sentinel node or nodes are negative, the patient can be spared axillary dissection. This technique is minimally invasive, and the accuracy of identification of the sentinel node or nodes is very high.

### Mastectomy

For eighty years, the radical or modified radical mastectomy was the treatment of choice for breast cancer, regardless of type, size of tumor, or patient's age. Breast conservation was not widely considered during this time. But, with recent advances in surgical procedures, less disfiguring operations can be performed. The days of the radical mastectomy, which removed the entire breast including the nipple and some lymph nodes under the arm as well as chest muscle, are gone. Surgical resection can be accomplished with minimal surgery without compromising long-term survival. Surgical oncologists now have several options from which to choose.

- The *modified radical mastectomy* removes the breast but does not remove chest muscle. Swelling of the arm because of removal of the lymph nodes may result in some patients.
- The *simple mastectomy* removes only the breast tissue including the nipple. No chest muscle is removed, and underarm lymph nodes remain, so arm swelling is reduced. But, if the cancer has spread to the underarm lymph nodes, it may remain undiscovered.
- *Lumpectomy*, known also as breast-conserving surgery, has received a lot of attention primarily because it is less invasive and disfiguring. This surgical procedure removes the tumor as well as a rim of tissue to make sure all cancer cells have been removed. Most of the breast is preserved. Clearly, size of the tumor is a factor in the consideration of lumpectomy versus mastectomy.

While some instinctively might think that "more is better," that removing the breast would be better than the breast-conserving lumpectomy to "be sure" that all cancer cells were removed, research has shown conclusively that that is not necessarily so. A twenty-year follow-up of a randomized study comparing breast-conserving surgery with modified radical mastectomy for early breast cancer found the long-term survival rate to be the same. From 1973 to 1980, approximately seven hundred women with breast cancers less than 2 cm in diameter were randomly assigned to undergo modified radical mastectomy or lumpectomy followed by radiation. Findings showed that the rate of death from all causes was 41.7 percent in the breast-conserving group versus 41.2 percent in the modified radical mastectomy group. The rates of death from breast cancer alone were 26.1 percent in the breast-conserving group versus 24.3 percent in the modified radical mastectomy group. These results were not statistically significant.[2]

Another recently published study, also a twenty-year follow-up randomized trial, investigated the outcome for women who were treated with lumpectomy alone or with lumpectomy and postoperative radiation compared to women who were treated with mastectomy. Researchers sought to determine whether less-invasive surgery was as effective as more radical surgery for treatment of invasive breast cancer. In this study, women with invasive breast tumors that were 4 cm or less in diameter and with either negative or positive axillary lymph nodes (stage I or II breast cancer) were randomly assigned to one of the three surgical treatment groups (mastectomy, lumpectomy, or lumpectomy followed by radiation). Axillary nodes were removed regardless of the treatment assignment. Findings showed no statistically significant differences among the three groups with respect to disease-free survival or overall survival. There was no difference in the likelihood that the disease would subsequently spread; nor was there any difference in the breast cancer death rate. Radiation, however, did markedly reduce the chance of another cancer developing in the same breast. For example, the risk that a second cancer would emerge in the same breast was 40 percent in the women who had a lumpectomy without radiation and 14 percent in those who had a lumpectomy followed by radiation.[3]

These dramatic findings have led to a shift in attitude toward breast cancer surgical treatment. It was shown conclusively that mastectomy is not necessarily superior to breast-conserving surgery and that uniformly performing a mastectomy may not necessarily be the most appropriate treatment of choice. Lumpectomy followed by breast irradiation is now viewed as an appropriate treatment option and a clinically proven treatment option that should be offered to most women diagnosed with breast cancer. Not every woman will be an appropriate candidate for lumpectomy, however. It is important, for example, to consider the size of the tumor in relation to the size of the breast. Those with relatively small breasts and large tumors, for example, might want to consider mastectomy followed by reconstruction for a better cosmetic look.

For those women who undergo a mastectomy, breast reconstruction is an option for consideration. The objective of breast reconstruction is to provide symmetry of the breasts and to have the individual feel more comfortable about her appearance. Saline implants can be used to match the reconstructed breast to the opposite breast. Other procedures transfer skin and muscle to the chest area from other areas of the body to provide symmetry. Reconstruction will depend on the type of mastectomy performed, skin and muscle condition, breast size, and postoperative treatment. Some women elect to have reconstruction at the same time as their breast surgery while others elect to have it done later. Reconstruction postmastectomy is a very personal decision and one that need not be made at the time of breast surgery.

## Radiation Therapy and New Techniques

While breast cancer is most often treated initially with surgery, increasingly women are receiving additional treatment, or adjuvant therapy, in the form of radiation therapy, chemotherapy, or hormone therapy. Localized adjuvant treatment (i.e., radiation therapy) focuses on a specific part of the body while systemic adjuvant therapy (i.e., chemotherapy or hormonal therapy) acts on the whole body. The selection of the type of adjuvant therapy is based on patient characteristics such as age, ethnicity, tumor size, histologic type, hormone receptor status, and other biomarkers (measurable parameters in tissues, cells, or fluids).

The goal of radiation is to kill the cancer cells directly or shrink the size of the tumor with high-energy external beams. Radiation is most harmful to rapidly reproducing cancer cells and prevents these cells from reproducing. For certain types of cancer, radiation is the only treatment needed. For other types, it is used in conjunction with other treatment modalities such as surgery and drug treatment. Radiation therapy, too, can be beneficial for patients with advanced stages of breast cancer for relief of symptoms and for slowing the progression of the cancer.

Available data indicate that postsurgical radiation provides a survival advantage irrespective of the type of surgery (mastectomy or lumpectomy) in node-positive women as well as node-negative women.[4] Radiation therapy after surgery has been shown to improve overall survival rates as well as reduce local recurrences in postmastectomy patients. Randomized controlled trials comparing radiation therapy to no radiation therapy have shown that those who received the therapy had fewer local regional recurrence (LRR) of the cancer, which resulted in a significant improvement in the overall survival rate and in the disease-free survival rate after a follow-up time of twenty years.[5]

Controlling local regional tumor recurrence leads to an improvement in survival rates. There is also evidence that high-risk patients, particularly those who have four or more positive lymph nodes or have an advanced primary cancer, also benefit from radiation therapy. Researchers have found that postmastectomy radiation reduced LRR for all patients regardless of the number of nodes involved.[6]

Radiation postlumpectomy is often the treatment of choice for women who have undergone this type of breast-conserving surgery. The various postlumpectomy radiation regimens currently in use differ in total radiation doses, volumes of breast tissue treated, duration of treatment, and techniques of administration. Radiation therapy is generally administered to women who have received breast-conserving surgery primarily because several studies have shown that breast-conserving surgery without subsequent radiation therapy results in higher breast cancer recurrence rates. The long-term benefits of radiation postlumpectomy in terms of survival and event-free survival in women with early stage breast cancer can be substantial.[7]

Although radiation therapy has been shown to improve survival, not all patients may need whole breast radiotherapy. Brachytherapy refers to a technique in which radioactive "seeds" are implanted or delivered by catheter near the tumor site. This targeted and localized delivery of radiotherapy has been used to treat prostate cancer and now is being used for some breast cancer patients (early-stage breast cancer; those whose tumors are no more than 2 cm in diameter). MammoSite, for example, is a Food and Drug Administration approved balloon-like device with a catheter that positions therapeutic radiation directly into the cancer site. While long-term studies on MammoSite's effectiveness are still being conducted, this form of radiation therapy has been shown to be less costly and more efficient in delivering radiation than traditional radiation therapy. Initial clinical experience with the MammoSite breast brachytherapy applicator in women with early-stage breast cancer treated with breast-conserving therapy, for example, has been generally positive.[8] Women who have highly confined lesions and who have involvement of only three or fewer lymph nodes would be the best candidates for these techniques.

A study comparing women who had a lumpectomy and who received this new form of radiation therapy to those who received the traditional external beam radiation therapy found no statistical differences in rates of local recurrence nor any differences in rates of distant metastasis, disease-free survival, or overall survival. Brachytherapy following lumpectomy was just as effective as traditional radiation therapy and took days instead of weeks to complete.[9]

With advances in ultrasound, digital mammography, and magnetic resonance imaging (MRI) technologies, there are now other new opportunities to take a more targeted approach in breast radiotherapy. Reducing the amount of breast tissue irradiated may make it possible to administer larger doses of radiation for a shorter period of time without significant toxicity. By relying on computerized algorithms, a smaller area of the breast can be targeted. This localized radiotherapy and image-guided partial breast irradiation are options for some patients.

The potential benefits of postsurgery radiation therapy have to be weighed against the short- and long-term side effects of this therapy. Clearly the dose and frequency of radiation treatment will have an effect on an individual. Common side effects of radiation for breast cancer include fatigue, skin redness, burns, and skin pain. For some, the nearest arm may swell and develop impaired mobility as a result of the radiation treatments. New procedures that employ precise targeting of the radiation to reduce the exposure to the patient serve to limit side effects. Yet, given the consensus of the research findings, radiation therapy is an important and beneficial form of treatment for women with breast cancer.

## Chemotherapy (Adjuvant Systemic Therapy)

Chemotherapy, the treatment of cancer with drugs, is used in addition to surgery and/or radiation therapy in an effort to destroy dividing cancer cells and prevent them from multiplying. These agents are given intravenously or orally, and usually multiple combination of drugs are used. Chemotherapy drugs are divided into several categories based on how they affect specific chemical substances within cancer cells, which cellular activities or processes the drug interferes with, and which specific phases of the cell cycle the drug affects. Some work directly on DNA to prevent the cancer cell from reproducing. Some interfere with DNA growth. Depending on the type of cancer and how advanced it is, chemotherapy can be used to cure the cancer, to control cancerous growth, or to relieve symptoms (usually pain) that are caused by cancer. Sometimes chemotherapy is given before surgery to help shrink the tumor.

Chemotherapy has been shown to substantially improve the long-term, relapse-free, and overall survival in premenopausal and postmenopausal women with node-positive and node-negative disease. Adjuvant chemotherapy was first used successfully in breast cancer patients with affected lymph nodes, and evidence suggests that both node-negative and node-positive patients will benefit.[10] Standard practice is to administer chemotherapy to most women with lymph node involvement or with primary breast cancers larger than 1 cm in diameter (node negative and node positive). For women with node-negative cancers smaller than 1 cm in diameter, the decision to consider chemotherapy should be individualized. Patients with small, node-negative breast cancers with favorable histologic subtypes may not need adjuvant chemotherapy.

There are substantial quality of life side effects of chemotherapy treatment, including hair loss, nausea, vomiting, fatigue, and potentially toxic side effects. In addition, the psychological distress of undergoing chemotherapy can be substantial, but for most women who may experience psychological distress, in the majority of cases, symptoms usually resolve once treatment ends.

Studies testing high-dose chemotherapy for qualified patients to ascertain its superiority to standard chemotherapy have been undertaken. There are major risks involved with high-dose chemotherapy including damage to the bone marrow and the production of needed blood cells, which would require subsequent bone marrow transplantation or peripheral blood stem cell transplantation to help the body produce blood cells needed for survival. Of interest was determining whether higher doses of chemotherapy prevented or delayed the spread or return of breast cancer better or more effectively than standard doses of the drugs. Would high-dose chemotherapy help patients live longer? A recent study comparing outcomes for 605 women with breast cancer who had four or more positive lymph nodes at the time they underwent surgery were given either a single course of high-dose chemotherapy or conventional therapy. Findings showed that survival without relapse after five years was similar, regardless of the type of therapy received. Overall survival, too, was similar. The results indicate that high-dose chemotherapy, with its increased toxicity and cost, did not confer a benefit.[11]

Research continues to provide information about the best combination of adjuvant chemotherapy treatment strategies. Ongoing studies are focusing on the identification of molecular markers that could be used to predict which patients with early-stage cancer would be most likely to have the cancer recur. These individuals would benefit the most from chemotherapy, but at present, there is no reliable way to tell which women would survive anyway without the chemotherapy. Research also is under way to discover different genetic patterns of tumors and identify those that would spread throughout the body and those that would not. Identifying the particular genetic characteristic of the tumor would enable doctors to tailor drugs to attack the particular molecular mechanisms of the tumor as opposed to the scatter-shot approach taken now.

## Hormonal Treatments

The growth of some breast cancers is sensitive or dependent on certain female hormones, estrogen in particular. Estrogen promotes the growth of breast cancer cells, but there are ways of medically blocking the effects of estrogen on these cells. Basically, hormonal therapies are designed to control the growth of hormone receptor positive breast cancer cells either by (1) blocking the receptors, (2) lowering the hormone levels, or (3) eliminating receptors. Breast tissue is analyzed to determine if the cancer cells have estrogen or progesterone receptors. The more estrogen receptors that are present, the more likely that antiestrogen therapy would be effective. The theory is that if there were less estrogen in the body, the hormone receptors would receive fewer growth signals so that cancer overgrowth can be stopped or controlled. Approximately 60 percent of breast cancers are estrogen-receptor positive. Antiestrogen therapy is not as effective in cancers that have few if any estrogen receptors.

Those individuals whose cancers are progesterone-receptor positive may also respond to antiestrogen therapy. If both estrogen and progesterone receptors are present, the chance of responding to antiestrogen therapy is high (70 percent). Those who are estrogen-receptor positive only or progesterone-receptor positive only have just a 33 percent chance of responding to antiestrogen therapy. If neither receptor is positive, the odds of responding to this therapy are quite low (10 percent).[12]

Over the years, there have been remarkable advances in hormonal therapies to treat breast cancer. Drugs designed to block the effects of hormones or lower the hormonal levels in the blood have increased the survival of women whose breast cancer is hormone dependent. Selective estrogen receptor modulators (SERMs) are powerful agents that act against the effects of estrogen in breast tissue, but also act like estrogen in other tissues. Probably the best known SERM is tamoxifen (brand name Nolvadex), which has been used in the treatment of breast cancer since the early 1970s and has been taken by millions of breast cancer patients. It is used as an adjuvant therapy following primary treatment for early stage breast cancer.

Tamoxifen (an antiestrogen), taken in pill form, interferes with the activity of estrogen by blocking the effect of this hormone in the breast tissue and slowing tumor growth. Yet, it acts like estrogen in other tissues of the body, which means it provides beneficial effects such as lowering blood cholesterol and reducing bone loss. When tamoxifen is taken as adjuvant therapy for early-stage breast cancer, it reduces the risk of recurrence of the original cancer and also reduces the risk of developing new cancers in the other breast.

Tamoxifen has been studied widely, most notably by the National Cancer Institute–funded Breast Cancer Prevention trial conducted by the National Surgical Adjuvant Breast and Bowel Project (NSABP), a clinical trials cooperative group formed in 1971 and supported by the National Cancer Institute. The NSABP's breast cancer studies led to the establishment of lumpectomy plus radiation over radical mastectomy as the standard surgical treatment for breast cancer. It was also the first to show that adjuvant therapy could alter the natural history of breast cancer, increasing survival rates as well as the first to show the preventive effects of tamoxifen in breast cancer.[13] The Breast Cancer Prevention trial, which included more than 13,000 women, showed the value of tamoxifen in reducing the incidence of breast cancer. Findings showed an almost 50 percent decrease in the diagnosis of invasive breast cancer in women at increased risk for the disease who took tamoxifen, in comparison to those who received a placebo, as well as a 50 percent reduction in the diagnoses of noninvasive breast tumors such as DCIS.[14]

Naturally, the benefits of tamoxifen alone or plus radiation therapy will vary with respect to the individual's disease status. Based on a model used to compare outcomes for hypothetical groups of postmenopausal women with estrogen receptor-positive tumors that are 2 cm or less in size with uninvolved axillary lymph nodes, however, studies indicate that recurrence-free survival rates were greater for those who were treated with tamoxifen plus radiation therapy versus tamoxifen alone after breast-conserving surgery.[15]

There are side effects of tamoxifen therapy similar to the symptoms of menopause (hot flashes, vaginal discharge or dryness) as well as more serious side effects (development of endometrial cancer and an increased risk of blood clots). Some women may experience irregular menstrual periods, headaches, fatigue, nausea and/or vomiting, cataracts, and skin rash; but, not all women who take tamoxifen will have any, some, or all of these side effects. Tamoxifen does not cause a woman to begin menopause, and in premenopausal women who are taking tamoxifen, the ovaries continue to produce estrogen in the same or slightly increased amounts. A five-year course of treatment is suggested for early-stage breast cancer patients, although individuals with advanced breast cancer can take the drug for varying lengths of time depending on their response to the medication.

Another SERM that is often prescribed is raloxifene (brand name Evista), originally developed to prevent and treat osteoporosis. Raloxifene works like an estrogen to stop bone loss and does not stimulate the breast or uterus as estrogen does. It lowers the blood concentrations of total and low-density lipoprotein cholesterol, although it does not increase the concentrations of high-density lipoprotein cholesterol (the good cholesterol). Because of its mechanism, it seems to have fewer serious side effects compared to tamoxifen. The most common side effects of raloxifene are hot flashes and leg cramps, and it is also associated with an increased risk of blood clots, but not endometrial cancer. The Food and Drug Administration has labeled raloxifene to be prescribed for the prevention of osteoporosis, but its effects on fracture risk and its ability to protect against cardiovascular disease needs to be determined. This drugs effect on breast cancer, too, is being studied, but the FDA has not approved it for breast cancer prevention at this time.

The Study of Tamoxifen and Raloxifene (STAR) clinical trial is designed to assess the effectiveness of both drugs. Over 19,000 postmenopausal women at high risk for breast cancer will be studied over a five-year time period. This is the first trial to compare a drug proven to reduce the chance of developing breast cancer (tamoxifen) with another drug that has the potential to reduce breast cancer risk (raloxifene).[16]

Results from the Multiple Outcomes of Raloxifene Evaluation (MORE) trial, designed to study raloxifene as a preventive agent for osteoporosis in postmenopausal women who were at high risk for this disease, showed a reduction in the incidence of breast cancer among study participants. After four years, women who took raloxifene had a 59 percent lower risk of breast cancer compared to those taking the placebo. The drug was especially effective in women with breast tissue that was sensitive to estrogen (estrogen-positive breast tumors).[17] Whether this finding will be true for other women remains to be tested.

Pharmaceutical research and development has led to the discovery of other powerful drugs shown to be somewhat successful in treating advanced breast cancer. Estrogen receptor down regulators (ERDs) are a new type of hormonal treatment for breast cancer that destroys receptors so that they cannot receive any more growth messages. In addition to binding to and blocking estrogen receptors, EDRs also stop or slow down the growth of breast cancer cells by breaking down the receptors. Faslodex, for example, is an ERD that has been approved for treating hormone receptor positive metastatic breast cancer in postmenopausal women with cancer that is no longer responding to hormonal therapy such as tamoxifen.

Another way to control the growth of hormone receptor-positive breast cancer cells is to lower the hormone levels using aromatase inhibitors (Arimidex, Femara, and Aromasin, for example). Aromatase inhibitors lower the amount of estrogen produced outside of the ovaries, thus blocking estrogen's ability to "turn on" cancer cells. Limiting the amount of estrogen that can be produced means that there is less estrogen available to reach cancer cells and promote growth. These drugs are used primarily for postmenopausal women with metastatic breast cancer.[18] Results from the Arimidex and Tamoxifen Alone or in Combination (ATAC) trial, a large-scale double-blinded randomized clinical trial, found that Arimidex is better than tamoxifen in postmenopausal women diagnosed with early-stage estrogen-receptor positive breast cancer and/or progesterone-receptor positive breast cancer. Arimidex reduced the risk of breast cancer recurrence by 17 percent more than tamoxifen alone and decreased the chances of breast cancer developing in the other breast by almost 80 percent.[19]

A recent double-blinded, placebo-controlled trial to test the effectiveness of five years of Letrozole therapy in postmenopausal women with breast cancer who had completed five years of treatment with tamoxifen was halted midway because of the startling difference in disease-free survival between the groups. The thinking was that the aromatase inhibitor, Letrozole, by suppressing estrogen production, could or might improve disease-free survival after the discontinuation of tamoxifen therapy. The results were so compelling that the study was halted after 2.5 years before the planned five years of study so that the new treatment could be made available to cancer survivors. When compared to placebo, Letrozole cut the recurrence rate nearly in half.[20] The issue of what to recommend after tamoxifen therapy is an important one, because post-menopausal women with hormone-receptor positive breast cancer are by far the most prevalent among breast cancer patients.

Despite the dramatic findings, many scientists expressed concern that halting this study midway made it impossible to answer important questions such as: Does Letrozole promote actual survival? How long should women take the drug? Does this treatment actually save lives? What are the long-term adverse risks of this treatment? What are the consequences of long-term use? There are several ongoing international trials studying the optimal duration and sequencing of treatment with tamoxifen and aromatase inhibitors, but the results will not be available for several years.

In summary, Tamoxifen, Faslodex, Arimidex, and aromatase inhibitors are hormonal therapies that interfere with the binding of estrogen in different ways. Although long-term effects of aromatase inhibitors are not known, trials such as the Arimidex, Tamoxifen, Alone or in Combination Trial will add to the body of knowledge and help tailor treatment options. For those who have contraindications to Tamoxifen, there are viable options.

## Biological Therapy (Immunotherapy)

Just as one's immune system defends the body against infections, it can also be the body's natural defense against cancer. New biological therapies use naturally occurring, normal proteins to repair, stimulate, and increase the body's ability to fight infections and cancer. These therapies boost the substances produced naturally by the body's own cells. HER-2 (human epidermal growth factor receptors) is a protein found to be a key component to regulating cell growth. When altered, extra HER-2 receptors may be produced, and this overexpression of HER-2 causes increased growth and reproduction, often resulting in more aggressive breast cancer with significantly shortened disease-free periods and survival rates. Approximately 25 percent to 30 percent of breast cancer patients are affected by HER-2 protein overexpression.[21]

Herceptin has shown promise in treating advanced breast cancer. This drug works only against breast cancers that make too much of the HER-2 protein. A landmark trial showed Herceptin's ability to increase patient survival time when compared to standard chemotherapy in patients with metastatic breast cancer that overexpresses HER-2. There are some serious side effects of this drug, however.[22] Herceptin can be cardiotoxic;

therefore, those who take the drug should have their heart monitored before and during treatment. Other less serious side effects include fever, chills, weakness, diarrhea, and nausea.

## Peripheral Blood Stem Cell Transplantation

It had been thought that high-dose chemotherapy followed by bone marrow or stem cell transplant was a promising treatment for some women with metastatic breast cancer. Stem cell transplantation involves the removal of stem cells from a patient's blood prior to treatment with high-dose chemotherapy. The stem cells are frozen and stored and then reintroduced intravenously after the chemotherapy ends. The protected stem cells can then begin to grow and produce different types of blood cells that the patient needs to survive. Clearly, there are major and serious risks involved with this procedure, and it may not be appropriate for everyone. Some studies on this type of treatment showed no clear benefit over the conventional and less aggressive treatments available. While one study found improved survival among women with widespread cancer, another found that although the treatment increased time to cancer recurrence, it did not improve overall survival rates.[23] At this time, peripheral blood stem cell transplantation is generally not recommended as a treatment option.

## New Techniques on the Horizon

New approaches to treating breast cancer focus on ablation of small tumors. Cryoablation targets small, minimally invasive tumors by means of insertion of an ultrasound-guided electric probe into a tumor. The tip of the probe is chilled with argon gas to form an ice ball around the tumor, and cycles of freezing and thawing are conducted to effect tumor cell death. Cryoablation therapy can be performed without general anesthesia or sedation and can be done in the office with the patient sitting up. Radiofrequency ablation, similar to the focused ultrasound, uses heat to destroy the tumor cells. In this therapy, an ultrasound-guided electrode probe is inserted into a tumor and another, larger electrode pad is placed on the skin surface. As the ions in the tissue try to follow the high-frequency current between electrodes, the tissue heats up and cells are killed. This technique is effective in treating small, primary breast tumors.

## RISK FACTORS FOR RECURRENCE

Surviving breast cancer depends on a woman's risk for return of cancer after treatment is completed. Some women are at higher risk for the return or spread of cancer, although the reasons for this are not clear. It is difficult to explain why one patient stays cancer free after treatment while another does not. There are several factors that probably contribute to recurrence: (1) tumor size: the smaller the tumor, the lower the risk; (2) lymph nodes: the fewer underarm lymph nodes that have cancer cells in them, the lower the risk; (3) cell growth: cancer cells that grow slowly and are less aggressive are linked to lower risk; (4) hormones: hormonal therapy can lower the risk of cancer spread or recurrence if the original tumor depends on hormones for growth.

For those who believed that performing a mastectomy would decrease the likelihood of recurrence, the findings from two large-scale, long-term studies clearly showed that there is no increased risk of recurrence if a lumpectomy is performed. The studies also showed that the incidence of recurrences in the node-positive women who received adjuvant chemotherapy was half the incidence in the node-negative women who did not receive that therapy. Clearly, size of tumor, nodal status, histological grade of the tumor, and a woman's personal risk factors will dictate not only the type of treatment but also the likelihood of cancer recurrence.

## SUMMARY

In November 2000, a panel of national and international experts at the National Institutes of Health (NIH) Consensus Development Conference on Adjuvant Therapy for Breast Cancer made recommendations about breast cancer treatments for all women. These recommendations included chemotherapy for most premenopausal and postmenopausal women with localized breast cancer, hormone therapy (most commonly with tamoxifen) for most women whose breast tumors contain estrogen receptors, and radiation therapy after surgery for all lumpectomy patients and some mastectomy patients who have large tumors or if four or more lymph nodes are found to be cancerous.

With the advances in early cancer detection and treatment, the prognosis for most women diagnosed with breast cancer is excellent. The earlier the cancer is detected, the better the chances of recovery and survival. The treatment options are constantly changing, and ongoing clinical trials are providing empirical data on a host of ways to fight breast cancer. The National Cancer Institute's Cancer Information Service can provide more information about breast cancer treatment clinical trials. However, there is no treatment option that is the "right" one. Treatment will vary depending on a number of factors including the cancer type, its stage, the tumor size and location, how fast it is growing (lab tests can measure how fast the cancer cells are dividing and how different they are compared to normal breast cells), lymph node involvement, whether the tumor is found to be dependent on hormones, an individual's age and menopausal status, and individual's overall health status. Also, almost all of the adjuvant therapies have short- and long-term side effects, some quite serious. Therefore, each individual must weigh the risks and benefits before deciding on one or more treatment modalities.

The diagnosis of breast cancer is not an automatic death sentence. Most women who are treated for early breast cancer go on to live healthy and active lives. My mother lived over fifteen active years after her mastectomy and chemotherapy. In fact, postmastectomy, and in her early sixties, she climbed not only the Himalayas but also the Peruvian Andes. In her late sixties, when her cancer recurred, she underwent another round of chemotherapy. Refusing to let her disease get the best of her, she managed to hike in the ruins of Petra (Jordan) with her daughter and granddaughter in between chemotherapy treatments!

## WEB SITES FOR FURTHER INFORMATION

http://www.breastcancer.org
http://www.nci.nih.gov
http://imaginis.com
http://www.thecancer.info/breast
http://www.breastdiseases.com
http://www.cancerquest.com

## CHAPTER 4

# The Principles of Cancer Screening and Diagnosis

Wﾠhile most of us are generally healthy most of the time, it is likely that serious disease will strike at some point in one's life. The biological onset of a disease occurs subclinically (a predisease stage such as an alteration in DNA, for example), and this stage usually precedes symptoms, which can occur months or years before one realizes that the disease is present. Breast cancer is a prototypical example of a progressive disease. As with most neoplasms, a breast cancer is believed to begin as a single malignant cell that grows rapidly and forms a proliferating tumor. Over time, breast cancer cells, if not destroyed, can spread through the lymphatic system to the axillary lymph nodes and eventually to other parts of the body via the lymphatic system, the vascular system, or both. Since breast cancer develops well before any signs or symptoms of the disease are noticed, it is difficult to pinpoint when the disease actually started.

There are several stages of disease progression. During the preclinical stage, when the disease has begun but is still asymptomatic, early detection followed by treatment could make a difference in disease progression and prognosis. The preclinical phase ends when the individual seeks medical attention because the symptoms have become apparent. Disease development then has moved from the preclinical stage to the clinical stage.

In order to make a diagnosis, a physician will perform an examination and order diagnostic tests to confirm a disease. Based on the medical findings, appropriate treatment is initiated. Most diseases can be treated successfully, returning the individual to a healthy, cured state (with or without disability). In some instances, the patient will not be cured per se, but the disease can be managed by medication or therapy. The least desirable outcome following diagnosis and treatment is death. Logically, disease detected at its earliest stage offers a greater chance for cure or survival.

Early detection of asymptomatic disease by screening is an excellent means for diagnosis and treatment. Screening refers to the application of a test to individuals who are asymptomatic. The purpose is to distinguish among apparently well individuals those who may have the disease from those who probably do not. Screening also can be used to identify people who are at high probability of having asymptomatic disease or who have a risk factor that puts them at high risk for developing the disease by virtue of their employment, their genetics, or their ethnicity. Screening tests *detect but do not predict* disease, and they provide information only about the individual tested at that point in time.

The purpose of the screening test—be it a chest X-ray, or blood or urine assays, or a mammogram—is to distinguish between those with normal test results and those with abnormal test results. It is important to stress that the screening test itself does not diagnose illness. Those who test positive on a screening test are sent for further evaluation to determine whether they do in fact have the disease. A screening test is not a confirmation of disease.

While the main objective of any screening test is to identify a subgroup of people with asymptomatic disease, there are different possible secondary objectives that are specific to the disease in question. For cancer screening, the objective of the test would be to identify patients at an early, preclinical stage of the cancer so that treatment can be initiated and survival chances hopefully increased. Screening for high blood pressure or diabetes, for example, is intended to identify patients with symptoms so that treatment can be initiated in order to prevent future complications associated with those diseases. Screening for sexually transmitted diseases or for tuberculosis is intended to eradicate infection and prevent its spread.

Another goal of screening is to reduce morbidity and mortality. Ideally, disease-specific death among those screened should occur at a lower rate than that for the general population. A common method of assessing the benefits of screening is to compare the five-year survival among screen-detected cases to that of the five-year survival of cases diagnosed at the clinical stage. All things being equal, there should be longer survival among screen-detected cases.

## WHAT CONSTITUTES A GOOD SCREENING TEST?

The first rule of thumb in screening for disease is that the disease must have the potential to result in significant morbidity or mortality. If the disease, left undiagnosed, does not produce significant morbidity or mortality, there is no compelling reason to screen for it. There is no point in screening for a disease that cannot be detected before symptoms appear. In fact, not every serious disease is appropriate for screening. Furthermore, there has to be an effective therapy for the disease once it is detected. A screening test that detects a disease in the presymptomatic stage is of little value unless there is effective treatment that could lead to a cure or increased longevity. If there is no effective therapy once the disease is detected, there is no value in screening. For example, screening for pancreatic cancer is not done because, while a serious disease, there is a slim chance of a cure or for long-term survival. For screening to be beneficial, treatment given during the preclinical or early stage of the disease should result in a better prognosis than therapy given after symptoms develop or after the disease is diagnosed at a later stage. If early treatment is not especially helpful or will not make a difference in the overall prognosis, then there is little value in screening.

In addition to the disease being serious and treatable, the incidence and prevalence of the disease should be high. If the disease were rare or uncommon, economically it would not be an appropriate disease for screening. One exception, for example, is screening newborns for phenylketonuria (PKU) because the test is inexpensive and the benefits of discovering even one case is high. PKU is a rare congenital metabolic disorder, which if left untreated leads to severe mental retardation. A simple urine test can detect this disorder, and if a newborn tests positive, intervention can begin soon after birth. The availability of a simple, accurate, and inexpensive test to detect PKU has led many states to require PKU screening for all newborns.

An effective screening test should ideally be inexpensive, easy to administer, and acceptable to the individual. Screening for high blood pressure, glaucoma, diabetes, or cholesterol levels includes tests that are quick, easy to administer, safe, acceptable, inexpensive, and effective. Screening for colon cancer, too, meets most of the above criteria; however, the screening test (either a sigmoidoscopy or colonoscopy) is not viewed as something pleasant to undergo nor is the cost inexpensive. As such, many individuals would prefer not to be screened for colon cancer by these means.

A good screening test should make a difference in prognosis and survival. That is, by screening and detecting disease at an early stage and by initiating treatment promptly for those whose disease is confirmed by further testing, these individuals should have a better prognosis because their disease was detected at an early stage. Screening for cervical cancer is an excellent example. If undetected and untreated, cervical cancer has a high mortality. The Papanicolaou smear test can detect precancerous cells, which can be surgically removed. The test is reliable, not terribly costly, easy to administer, and widely accepted by women. Those with cervical cancer who are treated at an early stage have an excellent prognosis. Those who are left untreated do not.

Implicit in any screening test is that treatment must be available for those who were screened and tested positive for the disease. Anyone who tests positive must receive a further diagnostic workup to rule in or rule out actual disease. It would be ethically incorrect and medically wrong to inform someone that he or she tested positive for a potentially serious disease and then not follow up with treatment.

In summary, a good screening test must be able to detect a potentially serious disease that many people have the potential to develop. The test must detect disease prior to clinical presentation. The disease should be more treatable when detected at an early stage, and there should be effective treatment available to those who are diagnosed with the disease. The test should be cost beneficial and easy to conduct on a large population. The test must be acceptable to those undergoing the screening process. While the criteria for a good screening test is somewhat straightforward, deciding on who should be screened is not.

## WHO SHOULD BE SCREENED?

Screening programs often take place in community settings such as in a shopping mall, at "health fairs," or at local health centers. Although such screening provides the opportunity to educate the public about disease and health, those who elect to be screened are self-selected. That is, these individuals are not only concerned about their health and well-being, but also are willing to be screened. For those who are told that their test result is abnormal, the individual would need follow-up testing to confirm that disease is present. It is important to reiterate that a screening test result is not a confirmation of disease. Given that there is usually no referral process for those who test positive at screening fairs, the onus is on the individual to make his or her own arrangements for further testing. Screening programs that take place at the local hospital or at one's doctor's office have the advantage of referring those individuals who test positive to the appropriate physician for further workup.

Figuring out who should be screened is best determined by deciding who would benefit the most from being screened. Just as it is neither practical nor logical to screen for every disease, one need not conduct mass screening on everyone in the population. Not only would this strategy be costly, not everybody is at equally high risk for developing disease. If the objective of a screening test is early detection, it is more sensible and cost effective to target cohorts who are at higher risk for developing the specific disease.

Targeting specific occupational groups or populations that have a known risk factor or are genetically susceptible to a disease is a common practice in disease screening. One would not screen the general population for carpal tunnel syndrome, for example, but one could initiate a screening program among assembly-line workers, individuals who are known to be at higher risk for this disease. Screening for Tay-Sachs disease among Ashkenazi Jews or sickle cell anemia among African Americans is more effective than mass screening for these diseases because these population groups are known to be at higher risk for these respective diseases.

## HOW "GOOD" IS THE SCREENING TEST?

Any screening test must be valid, reliable, and reproducible. The validity of a screening test refers to its ability to do what it is supposed to do. That is, the test must be able to categorize correctly individuals who have preclinical disease (test positive) and those without preclinical disease (test negative). Those who test positive for disease who actually have the disease are called "true positives." The test correctly identifies that disease is present. Those who test negative who do not have the disease are called the "true negatives." The test correctly indicates that no disease is present. Conversely, there are times when the test will be positive but the individual does not in fact have the disease. This group is referred to as the "false positives." Given that the test showed disease, albeit incorrectly, these individuals would be referred for further workup to rule in or rule out disease. Likewise, there will be times when a test shows no disease (negative test) when in fact the individual does indeed have disease. This group is referred to as the "false negatives." Given that the test showed no disease, even though disease is present, no further follow-up would be recommended. In a sense, the diseased individual would be given a false sense of security that he or she is well when in fact disease is present.

The false-positive group would undergo additional tests. The costs, discomfort, and anxiety associated with further testing are an unfortunate by-product of the screening test. The false-negative group, however, would have been told that the screening test showed no disease. For those who underwent mammogram screening and were told no disease was found when in fact cancer is present, a delay in treatment could be potentially disastrous. There are very few screening tests that correctly identify those with disease 100 percent of the time. Each test has some degree of margin of error, but that margin should be minimal.

Sensitivity and specificity are two measures of the validity of a screening test. Sensitivity the probability of testing positive if the disease is truly present. The specificity of a test the probability of screening negative if the disease is truly absent. A highly sensitive test will reduce the number of people who are incorrectly classified as false negatives. A highly specific test will reduce the number of people who are incorrectly classified as false positives.

Clearly, it is desirable that any screening test be both highly sensitive and specific to minimize misclassification. Unfortunately, this is usually not possible, and there must be a trade-off between sensitivity and specificity. A screening test that has the ability to avoid missing a true-positive case will do so at the expense of an increase in the number of individuals without the disease who will erroneously test positive. Deciding at what point a test result is considered normal or abnormal is a judgmental decision. Making less stringent the criterion of what is positive (high sensitivity) will mean that more people who have the disease will test positive. But, it also will result in an increase in false positives. Making more stringent the criterion for positive result (increased specificity) will mean that a greater proportion of those who test negative will actually not have the disease, but a greater number of true cases would be missed (decreased sensitivity). So, tests can be very sensitive but nonspecific or nonsensitive but very specific.

Which is better: to have a highly sensitive but less specific test or the other way around? Essentially, one has to weigh the consequences of leaving cases undetected (false negatives) versus erroneously classifying healthy persons as diseased (false positives). If a highly contagious disease is being screened, for example, and if the risk of missing a case is high because disease can be spread (AIDS or syphilis) or when subsequent diagnostic evaluations of positive screening tests are associated with minimal costs or risks (hypertension), it generally is preferable that sensitivity should be increased at the expense of specificity. If, however, the costs or risks associated with further diagnostic techniques are great (breast cancer), specificity should be increased relative to sensitivity.

While sensitivity and specificity measure the ability of a test to identify correctly diseased and nondiseased individuals, the reliability of a screening test refers to the consistency of results when repeated examinations are performed on the same persons under the same conditions; that is, the capacity of giving the same result (positive or negative, correct or incorrect) on repeated applications. While it is important that the screening machine or instrument be calibrated, human factors such as errors in interpretation of results may affect reliability. There may be differences in repeated measurements by the same screener, and there may be differences in interpretations of test results. Those conducting the screening must be trained in the same way, and multiple readings may be necessary to obtain accurate test results. Even with these safeguards, misinterpretations, mistakes, and misclassifications unfortunately occur.

While reliability does not guarantee high sensitivity and specificity, an unreliable test will not be sufficiently sensitive or specific to be useful. Yet, a test that is highly sensitive must be highly reliable when applied repeatedly to a diseased individual. Conversely, a test that is highly specific must be highly reliable when applied repeatedly to a nondiseased individual.

While sensitivity and specificity are characteristics of the test itself, it is important to take into account how prevalent the disease is. The practical value of a diagnostic screening test is dependent on the sensitivity, the specificity, and the disease prevalence. For a disease with a low prevalence (not many people have the disease), most of the population will be free of the disease, but of those who test positive (even for highly sensitive and specific tests) there will be a large proportion of false positives. Therefore, a good screening test should have a high predictive value (proportion of individuals who have a positive test really have the disease; proportion of individuals who have a negative test really do not have the disease). The predictive values of a test describe the frequency with which the results of the test represent correct identification of individuals as affected or not affected. For a disease of low prevalence, the predictive value of a positive test goes down sharply for the reasons just explained.

## DOES THE SCREENING TEST MAKE A DIFFERENCE?

The assumption that early detection will lead to longer survival is the basic premise of screening. The most definitive measure of the efficacy of a screening test is a comparison of the disease-specific mortality rates among those screened who had their disease detected early and those not screened who die of the disease. The best way to test this theory is to randomize people to screening versus nonscreening and see if there is a difference in rates of death from a specific disease. However, this experiment is not always feasible, practical, or ethical. When assessing survival among those screened, two concepts must be taken into account: lead-time bias and length bias.

Lead-time bias occurs when screening detects disease earlier than would have been detected due to development of symptoms, thus lengthening the time from diagnosis to death. It represents the amount of time by which the diagnosis has been advanced as a result of screening. Whether that lead time is days, months, or years will vary by the disease, the individual, and the screening test. If an estimate of lead time is not taken into account when comparing mortality among screened and unscreened populations, survival may mistakenly appear to be increased among those screened because the diagnosis was made at an earlier stage in the disease.

Length bias occurs when milder cases of the disease are detected disproportionately in population screening programs. More aggressive cases could have resulted in death or in symptoms requiring medical intervention without screening. Hence, those individuals screened may have a less aggressive tumor, for example, and are likely to survive longer regardless of the treatment given.

## MULTIPHASIC SCREENING

As the technology of screening has improved and as the costs of many screening tests have decreased, the reliance on multiphasic screening has increased. Multiphasic screening programs involve the screening for a variety of diseases at the same time in the same individual. Once a sample of blood has been drawn, for example, many different screening tests can be performed. Some organizations have developed proprietary lifetime health testing schedules whereby specific screening tests would be performed at specific ages from infancy to old age. These tests are directed toward conditions that have high prevalence at specific ages. For example, cervical cancer screening would be performed on younger and middle-aged women but probably not on older women. Prostate cancer screening would be performed on older men. Blood cholesterol levels would be performed at age-appropriate stages. Mammograms would be advised for women over age forty or fifty, depending on which guideline one follows.

The government has sponsored many large-scale screening programs. The Early and Periodic Screening, Diagnosis, and Treatment program is a federal–state program mandating access to health screening for Medicaid-eligible children under age twenty-one. The objective of this program is to improve children's health as well as to assess health needs to assure the early diagnosis and treatment of health problems. The emphasis is on preventive and primary care. Other large-scale government funded initiatives include: The Multiple Risk Factor Intervention Trial (MRFIT), which was funded by the National Heart and Lung Institute to assess the efficacy of a screening and intervention program directed against several risk factors simultaneously; and, The Veterans Administration Hypertension Detection and Follow-Up Program, which was designed to determine effectiveness of antihypertension therapy among individuals screened who were found to have elevated diastolic blood pressure.

In an effort to clarify issues concerning screening, the U.S. Department of Health and Human Services created the U.S. Preventive Services Task Force (USPSTF). The USPSTF is an independent panel of experts in primary care and prevention who systematically review the literature to develop recommendations for clinical preventive services. In the area of screening detection, for example, the panel's recommendations take into account not only the efficacy of screening tests in detecting disease, but also the extent to which early detection improves health. Multiphasic screening programs must guard against the failure to refer individuals who test positive for diagnostic follow-up.

## GENETIC SCREENING

The ability to perform quick, sensitive, and specific screening for genetic abnormalities or inherited tendencies is, to some extent, a reality. The Human Genome Project, whose objectives were to map the entire human gene system, has advanced knowledge of the genetic makeup of individuals. With this knowledge, there is the ability to identify individual genes and determine what they do and possibly, how they can be modified to treat or to prevent disease. The testing of an individual's genetic material to identify inherited risk for diseases can be used to confirm a suspected mutation in an individual or family. The potential impact on diseases treatment and prevention is immense.

The Office of Technology Assessment defines genetic testing as "the use of specific assays to determine the genetic status of individuals already suspected to be at high risk for a particular inherited condition." Genetic tests (biochemical, chromosomal, or DNA-based) need only be conducted once and are widely available for prenatal diagnosis of conditions such as Down syndrome, for example. They can identify cancer-related inheritable mutations in cells from tissue or blood in disease-free individuals. A negative test can create a huge sense of relief. It also may eliminate the need for frequent checkups and diagnostic tests. On the other hand, a positive test can also produce benefits by relieving uncertainty and allowing the individual to make decisions about medical treatment. Disease-free individuals who test positive for cancer-related mutations are candidates for primary preventive measures in hopes of preventing disease development.

Genetic screening, in comparison, is the systematic search of populations for individuals with latent, early, or asymptomatic disease. Such screening tests exist for breast and colon cancer, for example. Those who meet specific guidelines (personal medical history or member of a specific ethnic group in which the mutation is more common, for example) are good candidates for this testing.

Much of the current focus in gene testing centers on predictive gene testing; that is, tests that identify individuals who are at risk of a disease before any symptoms appear. In those cases in which a disease runs in the families, individuals who have a higher risk of inheriting a faulty gene could benefit by predictive gene testing. Unlike acquired mutations, heritable mutations confer an increased risk of disease. Hereditary cancers tend to occur at an earlier age than nonhereditary cancers, so at-risk individuals would benefit by being screened at a younger age. However, it is important to stress that a small percentage of the breast cancers detected in the United States are related to an inherited germline mutation usually in the BRCA1 or BRCA2 genes.[1] Hence, screening for BRCA mutations in the general population, and even among the majority of high-risk individuals, is probably not sensible. However, selective genetic testing offers an opportunity for individuals at hereditary risk for breast cancer to take proactive action regarding risk reduction and frequent surveillance.

Exciting research conducted at Memorial Sloan Kettering Cancer Center has followed 251 BRCA1 or BRCA2 mutation carriers who received genetic tests for breast and ovarian cancer between 1995 and 2000.[2] Two-thirds of the study population had mutations in BRCA1 and the rest in BRCA2. Each received genetic counseling as well as recommendations regarding available options for cancer screening and prevention. By offering options and support, these individuals who carried a potentially deadly gene were able to make difficult and emotional decisions. At the time of receiving genetic test results, 83.3 percent had breast tissue at risk, and 76.8 percent had ovarian tissue at risk. Patients were followed for a mean of 24.8 months. Twenty-one breast, ovarian, primary peritoneal, or fallopian tube cancers were detected after receipt of genetic test results. Many of the women elected to have risk-reducing prophylactic mastectomies and/or oophorectomies, and for several of these individuals, cancers were found in the tissue surgically removed. Genetic counseling and testing led to these risk-reducing operations, which resulted in the diagnosis of early-stage tumors in individuals with BRCA1 and BRCA2 mutations. Clearly, more research is needed to focus on the clinical and the psychological implications of genetic screening, but for those at high risk because they carry mutations in the genes BRCA1 and BRCA2, getting genetic counseling might help them make difficult choices. Each individual patient must weigh the risks as well as the benefits of genetic screening.

While tests for genetic screening create a host of personal choices/ decisions, the validity and utility of the genetic screening test must be taken into account. As with any screening test, it is important to assess a test's analytic validity (accuracy of the test to identify a DNA sequence variant), its clinical validity (accuracy with which the test predicts a particular clinical outcome such as breast cancer), and its clinical utility (the likelihood that it will lead to an improved health outcome).[3] Counseling patients and their family is imperative both before and after genetic screening. The potential benefits, limitations, and risks of genetic screening must be discussed. Deciding on which patients would benefit from genetic testing depends on the family history of cancer. Difficult questions associated with hereditary cancers require trained counselors' responses.

Predictive gene testing is exciting and potentially useful, but in most instances, the ability to initiate an intervention to prevent disease is not available. For example, predictive gene testing is available for approximately two dozen disorders including cystic fibrosis, Tay-Sachs disease, Huntington's disease, and for breast, colon, and thyroid cancers. But, the ability to actually prevent these diseases does not exist—yet. What is the clinician or the individual to do with the knowledge that the test shows a mutation in a gene sequence when there is no effective therapy to apply? What advice can one give an individual who has tested positive for Huntington's disease? There is no cure. There is no intervention.

Given the uncertainties of predictive genetic testing, ethical and psychological issues have to be addressed. A woman offered screening for BRCA1 and/or BRCA2 must understand the potential benefits of this test as well as the risks of knowing that she has this genetic mutation. Does an individual really wants to know the potentially worrisome truth if medical science cannot provide effective treatment or reassurance? What do the results mean for her? There are far-reaching consequences for an individual including reproductive decisions, lifestyle changes, and insurance issues.

Those involved in genetic testing, too, have difficult questions to answer. How should the results from predictive genetic tests be used? Who should have access to the test results? What options are there?

When should such a test be done—at what age? The Ethical, Legal, and Social Implications Program was established as an integral part of the Human Genome Project to look at the implications of these ethical issues.

Privacy and confidentiality issues need to be addressed more fully. Again, how should this new genetic information be used? Who should have access to it? How can individuals be protected from misuse of the information? Will test results become part of an individual's medical file, and what effect would the information have on insurability? One of the problems with reimbursement for genetic testing and counseling is that the insurance carrier would know that the test was performed. The insurance carrier might insist on knowing the results because it paid for the test.

## SUMMARY

Many screening tests—such as those for detection of hypertension, glaucoma, PKU, breast, cervical, and colon cancers are widely used. The objective is to detect disease in the preclinical stage, thus leading to early diagnosis and treatment, and hopefully to increased survival. Any good screening program must satisfy several specific requirements in order to be deemed appropriate. First, the disease should be associated with significant morbidity and mortality. If this requirement is not met, there is no point in screening. Assuming that the disease is considered serious, there must be effective therapy once the disease is diagnosed. Furthermore, the disease must be able to be detected in the preclinical, asymptomatic stage. The disease should not be rare, because screening would probably identify an unacceptable number of false positives, thus increasing the costs of further testing and increasing the anxiety for those who must undergo further testing.

Once one has decided that a disease would meet the requirements for screening, the screening test itself must be quick, easy, and inexpensive to administer. It must be safe and acceptable to those being screened. Most important, the sensitivity, specificity, and positive predictive value must be judged sufficiently high. Too many false-positive and false-negative test results are marks of a poor screening test.

Because screening tests identify those with abnormal test results, follow-up must be available. Those who test positive must be referred for further diagnostic testing and, if needed, treatment. There must be access to treatment. Ethically and medically, those who test positive cannot be abandoned at this stage. The treatment for the disease must be acceptable, otherwise those requiring treatment may not want to undergo it. Screening would have accomplished nothing. Above all, the test must do more good than harm. The benefits must outweigh the potential harms of testing healthy people.

Helpful questions for those undergoing a screening test:

- How "good" is the screening test? What is the sensitivity and specificity of the screening test?
- Is there evidence that early detection reduces morbidity and mortality?
- To what extent will I benefit if disease is detected early?
- What are the treatment options available in the event that I test positive?
- Do the medical benefits of screening outweigh the potential risks?
- What are the risks or possible side effects of the screening test?
- What are my options if it turns out that I am carrying a genetic mutation?

## CHAPTER 5

# Breast Cancer Detection: Old and New Techniques

Virtually all breast cancers arise from the glandular tissue. As such, it is important that these tissues are visible with as much resolution and contrast as feasible, within the constraints of low X-ray exposure. The discovery of the X-ray dates back to 1895, when the physics professor Wilhelm Roentgen, while working alone in his darkened laboratory, accidentally discovered "a new kind of ray." Not knowing what the emanations from his experiment were, he used the term X-ray to describe what he saw coming from his machine. The first X-ray picture was a radiograph of his wife's hand.[1]

Mammography is essentially a low dose X-ray of the breast used to detect changes. As early as 1913, a conventional X-ray machine was used to visualize breast cancers in mastectomy specimens, and mammography was first used in clinical practice in the late 1920s for the diagnosis of breast abnormalities.[2] Breast images were produced by standard X-ray machines, but the X-ray dose to the breast tissues was relatively high. Over the decades, the ability to diagnose breast tumors safely and accurately has become possible through dramatic advances in highly sophisticated imaging technology. In the 1960s, the dedicated first mammography machine was developed, and by the end of that decade, the first commercial model of the Senographe (French for "picture of the breast") was made available for commercial use. With further advances in imaging technology, screen-film mammography, which reduced the radiation doses, was introduced. In the 1970s, advancements in the technology allowed for a high degree of accuracy to differentiate between benign and malignant disease, making it more feasible for X-ray mammography to be widely used in breast imaging. Major improvements in the mammography equipment in the 1980s and 1990s further reduced the radiation dosage, improved the imaging, and reduced the effect of subject motion during exposure. Specifically, the first motorized compression mammography device was introduced in the early 1980s, which simplified mammography procedures. This advancement in the technology provided the impetus for mammography mass screening.[3]

## ENSURING QUALITY STANDARDS

In response to the proliferation of mammography facilities, there was a need for a breast cancer screening surveillance system. While the efficacy of mammography as a tool to screen and detect disease was being quantified, the safety of the units also needed to be documented. Prior to 1992, there were neither uniform standards to ensure that mammograms were safe and reliable nor uniform standards for technicians who perform the mammogram and physicians who read the film. States had varying quality control standards resulting in inconsistent and nonuniform readings. There were no record systems that could provide reliable and comprehensive data to permit the evaluation of the performance of screening mammography.

In an effort to set basic, minimum national standards, Congress enacted the Mammography Quality Standards Act of 1992 (MQSA). This act provided federal uniform quality control standards, instituted a system of inspection of mammography clinics, set training standards for technicians who perform mammography tests and for physicians who read mammography X-rays. It further required that women receive direct written notification of their results. The act stipulated that the FDA be responsible for accrediting and inspecting mammography facilities to certify that all facilities meet MQSA standards. Every facility is required to prominently display their FDA certificate.

A section of the MQSA authorized the establishment of a breast cancer screening surveillance system. In 1994, the Department of Health and Human Services was authorized to fund through the National

Cancer Institute the Breast Cancer Surveillance Consortium (BCSC), a consortium of research sites charged with assessing the effect of community mammography screening on stage distribution of breast cancer.[4] BCSC datasets are based on large populations drawn from diverse geographic and practice settings. As such, comparisons of regional data across the United States can be made.

In 1999, a revised ruling designed to strengthen standards relating to equipment to ensure that each unit is capable of producing high-quality mammograms took effect. The revised MQSA also required that mobile units be checked for acceptable performance each time the unit is moved to a new location and before any examinations are performed. As of 2001, there were 9,646 MQSA-certified mammography facilities in the United States and its territories.

There are occasional reports of shoddy mammography clinics in which either the quality of the film is poor or the interpretation of the film is substandard. In each of the last five years, more than 40 percent of the mammography facilities in the United States were cited for violating one or more federal rules.[5] While inspections are done primarily by the individual states, follow-up can vary tremendously. The FDA can levy fines of up to $10,000 a day to facilities in violation of federal rules, although it rarely does so. Clearly, those agencies that oversee the quality and safety of mammography facilities need to become more aggressive in their duty.

## USES OF MAMMOGRAPHY

It is important to distinguish between mammography as a screening tool and mammography as a diagnostic tool. For use in screening and detection, patients are presumably healthy and asymptomatic; individuals have no signs or symptoms of breast cancer. Mammography can detect microcalcifications (tiny deposits of calcium in the breast), which could indicate the presence of a tumor that cannot be palpated. Abnormalities that are detected by mammography require further examination.

A diagnostic mammogram is used to diagnose suspicious breast changes such as a lump, pain, thickening, or nipple discharge. It also is used to investigate changes detected on a screening mammogram. A diagnostic mammogram takes more time than a screening mammogram because it involves more X-rays to view the breast from several angles. There are some specialized mammography units designed for both screening and diagnostic images.

## EVIDENCE OF BENEFITS OF MAMMOGRAPHY

Several major studies provided the impetus for and feasibility of mammography screening. The groundbreaking Health Insurance Plan (HIP) of New York study (1963–1967) was one of the first and the largest mammography studies to be conducted. This randomized clinical trial of more than 60,000 women between the ages of forty and sixty-four showed that screening asymptomatic women for breast cancer could cut the breast cancer death rate significantly.[6] The study showed that, among those women aged fifty and older who had a mammogram there was a 25 to 30 percent reduction in mortality. That is, the breast cancer death rate was about 30 percent higher in women who did not have mammograms. Of the approximately 30,000 women who were not screened by mammography, 196 died of breast cancer compared to 153 of the approximately 30,000 women who were screened by mammography. It should be stressed that this study was initiated at a time when mammograms were not in general use. It was assumed that it would be unlikely that the women who were randomly assigned to forgo screening (they were not invited for mammogram screening) would not get a mammogram on their own. (See chapter 6 for a more complete discussion of this study.)

Inspired by the early reports of favorable results from the HIP study, the ACS proposed to the National Cancer Institute a collaborative effort to demonstrate the feasibility of large-scale screening for breast cancer.[7] The Breast Cancer Detection Demonstration Project (BCDDP) was conducted from 1973 until 1980 and followed over time 283,000 asymptomatic women between the ages of thirty-five and seventy-five. These women were screened annually for five years. Findings from a twenty-year follow-up show that mammography was very effective in identifying most cancers in all age groups, but was more sensitive in the older women. Mammograms did not detect 10 percent of cancers in women younger than fifty years of age compared to 5 percent in women older than age fifty.[8] Of the 4,443 cancers found, 42 percent were discovered by mammography and 8.7 percent by physical examination.

Very high survival rates for up to a decade were observed among the 4,240 women with a histologically confirmed diagnosis of breast cancer.

The relative five-, eight-, and ten-year survival rates were 88 percent, 83 percent, and 79 percent, respectively.[9] Researchers concluded that there was little doubt of the benefits of screening for breast cancer with mammography in both younger and older women. The shift toward a high proportion of cancers being diagnosed and treated at more favorable stages as a result of screening contributed to substantial gains in breast cancer survival.[10]

While more empirical studies were needed to validate the benefits of mammography among asymptomatic women, two major events in the mid-1970s did more to encourage women to undergo mammogram screening than anything else. Within a few years of each other, both the president's wife (Betty Ford) in 1973 and the vice president's wife (Happy Rockefeller) in 1974 were diagnosed with breast cancer, and both had a mastectomy. The tremendous publicity served to galvanize women to have a mammogram. While the findings from the prospective trials served to affirm the benefits of regular mammogram screening, it was the personal experience of Mrs. Ford and Mrs. Rockefeller, and their willingness to talk about their breast cancer and the importance of breast cancer screening, that provided the impetus for women to be screened.

## WHO IS MORE LIKELY TO HAVE A MAMMOGRAM?

After more than two decades of urging women to have regularly scheduled mammograms, it seems that few actually do so. In one of the most detailed and largest studies to quantify the extent to which women follow recommendations to have regular mammograms, researchers from the Harvard Medical School found that only 6 percent of women who received a mammogram in 1992 received mammograms yearly for the next ten years.[11] This finding was based on a study of over 72,000 women of all ages who received screening mammography at the Massachusetts General Hospital between 1985 and 2002. Only one in twenty women consistently followed the recommendations for annual mammograms. The study also found that among women diagnosed with invasive breast cancer, those who had prompt annual mammograms had a lower risk of death (approximately 12 percent) compared to those who received mammograms every two years (approximately 16 percent) or every five years (approximately 25 percent).

It is well known that poor women, those who do not have health insurance, those from nonwhite ethnic groups have particularly low rates of getting a mammogram. The Harvard-Massachusetts General study confirmed that women from lower SES got fewer mammograms than women who were more affluent. African American, Hispanic, and Asian women got fewer mammograms compared to white women. Furthermore, data collected by the BCSC from the years 1996 to 2000 showed that of the approximately 2.8 million mammograms recorded, two-thirds were performed on white, non-Hispanic women, while only 5 percent were done on black, non-Hispanic and 6.6 percent on Hispanic women. The data also show that of those who do get a mammogram, 40 percent of the women reported having only a single screening mammogram. Annual or biannual screening was not reported by most of the respondents.[12]

These findings are disturbing because as the following discussion illustrates, mammography, even with its flaws, is the best means of detecting early-stage breast cancer as a population-based screening program. While there are other methods to detect breast cancer, none are suitable as a means of mass screening.

## MAMMOGRAPHY: SENSITIVITY AND SPECIFICITY

While mammography screening remains the gold standard for detecting early-stage breast cancer, there are limitations of this procedure that need to be acknowledged. First, the sensitivity and specificity of mammography is not 100 percent. Estimates of sensitivity and specificity of mammography will vary with the methods used to calculate it.[13] Negative findings on a mammogram do not always rule out breast cancer, and positive findings do not always indicate malignancy. The overall sensitivity (ability to detect cancer when it is present) of screening mammography ranges between 71.1 and 91.5 percent. Among women older than age fifty, the sensitivity is between 85 and 90 percent. Sensitivity is lower among women younger than age fifty primarily because these women tend to have denser breasts, making it more difficult to detect cancer. While the sensitivity is fairly high, the specificity (ability to correctly identify those without cancer) is low. Ranges of specificity range from 30 to 65 percent. The specificity among younger women younger than age fifty is not as good as that for women over age fifty.

Although the estimates of sensitivity of mammography are variable (depending on patient characteristics and other factors), some of the explanations for this involve technical reasons and interpretation errors. Missed lesions could occur because of the radiographic technique (positioning of the patient, processing of the film) or because of poor-quality film. Poor-quality films can lead to mistaken diagnosis and misinterpretations of the film. Misinterpretations of the film, failure to detect a tumor, and misidentification of a tumor are some of the known problems with mammography.

Although mammography is a highly effective method of early detection of breast tumors, it is technically one of the most difficult radiographic investigations to interpret. Finding breast cancer is not always easy; a cancerous lesion can be seen on a mammogram only if it looks different from surrounding breast tissue. In some cases, the cancer is indistinguishable from normal tissue. The menstrual cycle also affects accuracy. Accuracy is more likely if menstruating women have a mammogram during the first or second week of the menstrual cycle when breast tissue is less dense, for example. Even the best radiologist does not have a 100 percent rate of detecting cancers on mammography, and physician variability in reading the films is well documented. Studies have shown, however, that if previous mammograms were available to the radiologist, the number of false positives would decrease. One study found that when the radiologist had access to the woman's previous mammogram, the incidence of false positive mammogram readings was reduced by at least half.[14]

## THE IMPORTANCE OF VOLUME: PRACTICE MAKES PERFECT

As is true with many things, the more films a radiologist interprets, the greater the likelihood that his or her skills will be perfected. Volume is an important factor in honing skills.[15] Countries with socialized medicine, such as the United Kingdom and Sweden, have adopted a centrally organized approach to screening. The result is high specificity (low percentage of false positives) and high sensitivity (high percentage of true positives). In contrast, the United States has a decentralized system that is not organized around high-volume centers. The annual reading volume for radiologists in the United States varies greatly and is much lower than that in either Sweden or the United Kingdom, for example.[16] The minimum annual reading volume in the United States is 480 as set by the MQSA of 1992; the minimum set by the National Health Service Breast

Screening Programme in the United Kingdom is an impressive 5,000 mammograms per year.[17]

Studies have shown that low-volume American radiologists and medium-volume American radiologists had statistically significantly lower sensitivity than British radiologists. Reader volume is a very important component and determinant of mammogram sensitivity and specificity, as radiologists who read a low volume of mammograms are less likely to interpret them accurately compared to those who read a lot of films.[18] Yet, reading large volumes of mammograms is only one factor affecting radiologists' accuracy. Some have questioned whether the volume of mammograms read, the number of years of experience reading mammograms, or even lifetime number of mammograms read should be used to determine the experience of a radiologist.[19]

## WHAT ABOUT FALSE POSITIVE AND FALSE NEGATIVE READINGS?

The proportion of all mammograms that are false positives (i.e., they suggest abnormalities that after further testing turn out to be benign) is higher than one might think. False positives are more common in younger women, women who have had previous breast biopsies, women with a family history of breast cancer, and women who take hormones. A large-scale ten-year study based on 9,762 screening mammograms and 10,905 screening clinical breast examinations found that of the women screened, one-quarter had at least one false positive mammogram, 13.4 percent had at least one false positive breast examination, and 31.7 percent had at least one false positive result for either test. Among women who did not have breast cancer, an estimated 18.6 percent undergo a biopsy after ten mammograms and 6.2 percent after ten clinical breast exams. Over ten years, one-third of the women screened had abnormal test results requiring additional evaluation, even though no breast cancer was present.[20]

The more mammograms a woman has, the greater the likelihood of a false positive reading. If a forty-year-old woman was screened annually for ten years, she would have a 30 percent chance of having at least one abnormal screening examination that would require a diagnostic workup, a 28 percent chance of at least one false positive exam, and a 7.5 percent chance of having a breast biopsy. Alternatively, a fifty-year-old woman having the same ten mammograms over ten years has a 26 percent

**Table 5.1**
**Risk of at Least One Abnormal Mammographic Exam, False Positive Exam, and Breast Biopsy If Screened Annually for Ten Years**

|  | Age | | | |
| --- | --- | --- | --- | --- |
|  | 40 | 50 | 60 | >70 |
| Risk |  |  |  |  |
| Abnormal exam | 30% | 26% | 23% | 26% |
| False positive exam | 28% | 23% | 20% | 22% |
| Biopsy | 7.5% | 10.4% | 10.4% | 10% |
| Invasive breast cancer | 1.5% | 2.4% | 3.4% | 3.5% |

*Source:* Kerlikowske, K and Barclay, J. Outcomes of Modern Screening Mammography. Journal National Cancer Institute Monographs 22:105–111. 1997.

chance of at least one abnormal screening exam, a 23 percent chance of having at least one false positive exam, and a 10.4 percent chance of undergoing at least one breast biopsy.[21] Table 5.1 shows the risk of at least one abnormal mammographic exam, false positive exam, and breast biopsy at different ages.

In addition to age, use of HRT increases the risk of false positive readings. Findings from the Million Women study in the United Kingdom clearly showed that use of HRT was estimated to have been responsible for 20 percent of the cases of false positive recall.[22] False positive recall was significantly increased in current and past users of HRT compared with never users, although the relative risk of false positive recall decreased significantly with increasing time since last use of the medication.

The burden of false positive readings has financial and emotional consequences. Additional testing will have to be done, and the anxiety of waiting for the results can take its toll on the woman and her family. While the number of false positive readings, fortunately, is only a small proportion of the total number of mammograms read, it should be understood that the probability increases by age of woman. However, the vast majority of false positive readings will turn out to be a false alarm. For example, among one hundred women aged forty to forty-nine who have an abnormal first screening, ninety-four will not have cancer. But, these women will have undergone further testing before breast cancer is ruled out. The cost of this additional testing in the United States is significant.[23]

## BALANCING MAMMOGRAPHY'S BENEFITS AND HARMS: OVERDIAGNOSIS

While the objective of breast cancer screening is to detect a cancer at its early stage, some cancers are so slow growing that failure to detect them would not make a difference in overall survival. To what extent does mammography screening increase the likelihood that these cancers are detected? Is it necessarily a good thing that these types of cancers are found? What are the consequences to the individual?

Overdiagnosis in cancer screening is defined as the detection of cancers that grow so slowly that they are unlikely to be diagnosed during a person's lifetime. Studies looking at the issue have provided evidence suggesting that overdiagnosis of invasive breast cancer occurs with screening mammography. Using breast cancer incidence rates in Norway and Sweden, researchers found that cancer incidence among women aged fifty to sixty-nine years increased substantially after the implementation of screening programs They concluded that one-third of all cases of invasive breast cancer in this study sample were overdiagnosed; that is, without screening, these cases would not have been detected during the individual's lifetime.[24] A host of factors could have contributed to this finding, of course, and estimating the true extent of overdiagnosis is difficult. But, it is important to raise the issue and help women understand the potential consequences of overdiagnosis such as unnecessary breast surgeries and treatment. Most would agree that the benefits of mammography outweigh the harms, but that the benefits may come at the cost of some over-diagnosis of breast cancer, which, if left alone, probably would not affect survival. Advances in precision and accuracy of screening technology are helping to permit a more precise diagnosis of suspicious lesions.

## ADVANCES IN BREAST IMAGING

In the recent past, women whose mammogram looked suspicious or abnormal had few follow-up options available. They were often instructed to return within six months for a follow-up mammogram. This "wait-and-see" approach not only would increase the anxiety of uncertainty, but also could jeopardize early detection and possibly lower the chance for survival if a malignant lesion is detected later. Detecting a cancer before it has spread to other parts of the body is the objective and purpose of new technologies. There are several highly sophisticated technologies that now permit a more precise examination of suspicious lesions. However, finding or detecting breast cancer does not necessarily translate into a life saved. Fast-growing or aggressive tumors that have already spread to other parts of the body before being detected, for example, are found "too late." In some cases, a mammogram would not have shown the tumor until it became apparent as a discernible lump. Recent developments in technology that include using magnets, sound waves, and cellular biology as screening tools have helped in the detection of some difficult to discern breast lesions. While mammography is still viewed as the gold standard for mass screening, these new technological advances have the potential to increase accuracy.

Whereas conventional mammography relies on an X-ray image of the breast tissue, which is then made into a printed image, new techniques utilizing complex computer systems have the ability to see tumors not visible on mammography. At this time, none of these technologies should serve as a replacement for mammography screening. They are, however, shown to be excellent adjuncts to mammography.

## Digital Mammography

Digital mammography uses X-rays to create an image of the breast on a computer screen. A detector responds to X-ray exposure and sends an electronic signal to a computer to be digitized and processed. Computer programs aid in the detection and characterization of breast masses and calcifications and allow the radiologist to adjust images to help detect subtle differences between tissues.[25] The first digital mammography system received FDA approval in 2000. The procedure for digital mammography is the same as that for conventional mammography. The images captured on digital mammography can be stored and retrieved electronically. There are no films to develop.

Digital mammography offers advantages over conventional mammography in that the digital image can be manipulated postprocessing; adjustments in brightness and contrast are possible, and selected areas of the breast can be electronically magnified, thus permitting the radiologist to adjust images to help detect subtle differences between tissues. Since the image is stored in a computer, the radiologist can send the image electronically to colleagues in other centers for a second opinion. While digital mammography has the ability to "see" more than conventional mammography, there are current limitations, including the prohibitive cost.

## Computer-Aided Detection

Computer-aided detection (CAD) uses the computer to highlight suspicious areas for more intense review, perhaps reducing the number of false positive results. The ImageChecker is an example of CAD technology.[26] This device scans the mammogram with a laser beam to create a digital signal. The image is displayed on the computer monitor, and any areas that the system regards as suspicious are highlighted. These suspicious areas can be viewed more carefully. This technique is particularly useful in cases that would ordinarily require a second reader because of suspicious findings. The CAD system is designed to assist the radiologist in reducing the number of false negative readings by focusing attention to areas that may warrant a second review. It is a fairly new technique, and it remains to be seen if CAD technology improves the accuracy of screening mammography. CAD used alone has very low specificity, which is a limitation.

Numerous studies are ongoing to assess CAD and to address the unanswered questions about the superiority of digital to conventional mammography. It is important to understand that whether conventional or digital mammography is used, the woman is still getting a mammogram. Whereas conventional mammography is sensitive and specific, sensitivity and specificity for CAD is not yet known for general screening populations. As research studies are completed, information on the benefits of digital mammography should be clearer.

## Ultrasound

Although not considered to be a useful population-based screening device per se, ultrasound technology can aid in the detection and diagnosis of breast disease. Ultrasound is the use of high-frequency sound waves to generate an image. Ultrasound imaging of the breast is used to distinguish between solid tumors and fluid-filled cysts. It also can be used to evaluate lumps that are hard to see on a mammogram, but ultrasound does not detect microcalcifications well (a cluster of microcalcifications may indicate that cancer is present). Ultrasound is an adjunct to mammography, particularly for the evaluation of dense breasts. At this point in time, it is not a suitable screening tool even though it is inexpensive and relatively quick. It usually is used as a follow-up to a suspicious mammogram and as part of other diagnostic procedures such as fine-needle aspiration or needle biopsy.[27]

While the sensitivity and specificity of ultrasound ranges from 85 to 97 percent (higher than that of mammography), there are several disadvantages to ultrasound as a screening tool. As mentioned previously, it has a poor ability to detect microcalcifications as well as ductal carcinoma in situ, which is often not seen on ultrasound. There are new ultrasound technologies in the early stages of development, which have the potential to overcome some of the drawbacks to conventional ultrasound. The high-frequency, hand-held devices can differentiate cysts from solid masses and provides guidance for core-needle biopsy and cyst aspiration. Real-time ultrasonography permits scanning of the maximum dimensions of the tumor as well as direct measurements without magnification. This allows for more accurate determination of tumor size.

## Magnetic Resonance Imaging

Magnetic resonance imaging (MRI) uses a magnet and radio waves to make a series of detailed pictures of areas inside the body. MRI does not use any X-rays. Rather, a magnet is linked to a computer to create detailed pictures of areas inside the body without the use of radiation. Hundreds of images of the breast are taken, which are then interpreted by the radiologist. A patient may be given a nonradioactive contrast agent intravenously to improve visibility because breast tumors show an increased uptake of the contrast agent. MRI of the breast depicts the size of a malignant mass more accurately than mammography among women at high risk of breast cancer, particularly in women with an inherited susceptibility to breast cancer.[28] MRI of the breast also can be effective for women with dense breasts, for women with breast implants to detect leaks or ruptures, or it can be used after breast cancer is detected to determine the extent of the tumor. It is used as well to diagnose fibroadenoma, a benign breast tumor most common among women younger than age thirty.

MRIs are more accurate than mammography in evaluating the actual size of a malignancy and thus helpful in establishing an appropriate treatment protocol. It also is a useful biopsy-guidance technique, but only if the lesions were detected with MRI. The MRI has a high sensitivity in the detection of breast cancer, but its specificity is relatively low.[29] While an MRI can distinguish benign tumors from malignant lesions quite accurately, it cannot detect microcalcifications. The consensus at this time is that even though MRIs might detect more tumors, they might also produce too many false alarms (false positives).

At this time, there are no standardized procedures for dose and timing for MRI of the breast. Radiologists would need training in MRI interpretation, and, to further complicate matters, there is a lack of uniform interpretation criteria. If MRI is to play a more significant role in breast cancer detection, the cost of the procedure will have to be addressed as well. At the present time, the high cost of an MRI as well as its limitations precludes its widespread use in breast cancer imaging.

## Scintimammography

The ability of mammography to detect breast pathology can be limited by the density of the breast tissue or the presence of fibrocystic breast change.[30] The objective of scintimammography (SMM) is to improve the sensitivity of detecting tumors in patients with suspected breast cancer. SMM, also called Technetium Tc99 Sestamibi breast imaging, involves the use of nonspecific, tumor imaging radionuclides in the diagnosis and staging of breast cancer. Patients receive a trace amount of a radiopharmaceutical by injection and are then imaged with a special gamma camera. There is no breast compression as with a mammogram or MRI.

SMM is used as a complementary diagnostic procedure when mammography results are suspicious; it is not indicated for breast cancer screening nor is it an alternative to biopsy. It is useful for patients with dense breasts; patients who have scarring or distortions of the breast due to previous breast biopsy or surgery, radiation therapy, or chemotherapy; and patients with breast implants. It could be considered an option for women with an abnormal mammogram to evaluate the lesion in greater, more precise detail, and aid in the confirmation of the diagnosis and early detection. It also has been shown to be useful in younger (younger than fifty years of age) and premenopausal women with suspicious breast lesions. In combination with mammography, SMM offers significantly improved sensitivity and accuracy in detecting breast cancer in premenopausal women, in women with dense breasts, and in women with hard to image breast tissue.[31]

Numerous studies have assessed the diagnostic accuracy of SSM. High sensitivity in the detection of palpable and nonpalpable breast lesions and for detecting cancer in patients with dense breasts has been shown.[32] The sensitivity and specificity of this imaging modality were at least the same or better than that for mammography. Radionuclide breast imaging should be considered an adjunct to current screening procedures especially among women with dense breasts, those with palpable abnormalities, and abnormal mammograms.

## Positron Emission Tomography Scan

Positron emission tomography (PET) scans create computerized images of chemical changes that take place in tissue. An injection of glucose containing a radioactive atom is administered. Cancer cells absorb radioactive sugar faster than other tissues in the body; if a tumor is present, the radioactive sugar will accumulate there. The PET scanner detects the radiation, and the computer translates the information into the images that are interpreted by a radiologist. PET scans are more accurate in detecting larger (>8 mm) and more aggressive tumors. They are helpful in evaluating and staging recurrent disease. Whole-body PET scans can identify metastatic breast lesions and may be useful in monitoring the effectiveness of chemotherapy in patients. There is high sensitivity (visualizing between 82 and 100 percent of primary tumors), depending on tumor size and other considerations. Data on specificity are not yet available.[33] Both the SMM and PET scans are expensive technologies. Neither is a cost-efficient screening tool; however, each can add value to diagnosing tumors not clearly delineated by mammogram.

## Breast Thermography

This diagnostic technique images the breast to aid in the very early detection of breast cancer.[34] Breast thermography is based on the principle that chemical and blood vessel activity in both precancerous tissue and the area surrounding a developing breast cancer is always higher than that for normal breast tissue. Precancerous and cancerous tumors need blood and other nutrients to grow, and their metabolic activity increases the surface temperature of the breast. An abnormal infrared image is the single most important marker of high risk for developing breast cancer; it is a potentially strong early warning sign.

Digital infrared imaging (DII), or breast thermography, uses ultrasensitive infrared cameras and sophisticated computers to detect, analyze, and produce high-resolution diagnostic images of temperature variations. These temperature variations are thought to be very early signs of breast cancer or precancer, which cannot be detected by other screening procedures. An abnormal infrared image is an important marker of high risk for developing breast cancer. In the absence of other positive tests, an abnormal infrared image gives a woman an early warning.

DII involves no radiation, compression of the breast, or intravenous contrast. Sensitivity and specificity are both estimated to be 90 percent.[35] Although the procedure can detect variations in blood vessel activity, thermography does not have the ability to pinpoint the location of a tumor. As such, it should be used in combination with, not instead of, mammography. Furthermore, it requires access to sophisticated technology and the expertise to interpret the findings.

## Electronic Impedance Scanning

Electrical impedance refers to the speed at which electricity travels through a given material. Tissues have different electrical impedance levels; for example, cancerous tissue has a lower electrical impedance than normal tissue—it conducts electricity much better. The device, unlike mammography, does not emit radiation nor does it require compression. An electrode patch is placed on the arm, and a small amount of electric current is transmitted through the patch into the body. The current travels through the breast and measured by the hand-held scanning device. An image is generated on a computer based on the measurements of the electrical impedance. Breast tumors appear as bright white spots on the computer screen because breast cancer cells conduct electricity better than normal breast cells and tend to have lower electrical impedance.[36]

Based on clinical trials evaluating safety and effectiveness, the T-Scan 2000, for example, was approved for use as an imaging device by the FDA in 1999. It is intended for use as a follow-up to mammography for those whose mammograms are suspicious. That is, the device can confirm the location of abnormal areas detected by mammography, thus perhaps reducing the number of biopsies needed to determine whether a mass is cancerous. The scanner is not an approved screening device for breast cancer, but is an excellent tool to use when more conventional tests indicate suspicious lesions. Electrical impedance scanning devices have been used with mammography to confirm the location of abnormalities. It is not recommended for use on patients who have implanted electronic devices such as pacemakers.

## Image-Guided Techniques

A variety of image-guided procedures are being used to supplement mammography for a nonpalpable abnormality discovered on a mammogram. The objective of image-guided procedures is to lead to more accurate characterization of breast masses and hopefully less surgery for breast cancer patients. Image-guided core-needle breast biopsy involves a stereotactic or ultrasound-guided procedure to permit the precise location of the abnormal area on mammography. Stereotactic refers to the use of a computer and scanning devices to create three-dimensional images.[37] A stereotactic needle biopsy guided by mammography is less expensive and less invasive than a traditional surgical excisional biopsy and results in less breast deformity.

## Ductal Lavage

Since the overwhelming number of breast cancers start in the epithelium lining the ductal system, looking for abnormal cells in the milk ducts is viewed as a good way for early detection. Ductal lavage is a procedure designed to collect efficiently breast epithelial cells for analysis.[38] This technique tests milk duct cells to detect atypical cellular changes within the breast tissue. A saline solution is introduced into a milk duct through a catheter inserted into the opening of the duct on the surface of the nipple. Fluid, containing cells from the duct, is withdrawn through the catheter. The cells are checked under a microscope to identify changes that might indicate cancer or precancerous changes that might increase the risk for breast cancer. It is approved for women at elevated risk for breast cancer. While safe and well tolerated, this procedure is not appropriate for population-based screening. The sensitivity and specificity of this procedure is not yet determined.

## Other Imaging Techniques

Some of the most recent technologies being tested have the potential of detecting cancer at an early, more treatable stage. New technologies on the horizon include: Magnetic Resonance Elastography, Electrical Impedance Spectroscopy, Microwave Imaging Spectroscopy, and Near Infrared Spectroscopic Imaging. These complex and highly sophisticated technologies try to identify changes associated with tumor growth. An endoscope that is less than 1 millimeter in diameter can be used to magnify breast tissue and pinpoint lesions. The endoscope is inserted through the nipple into the ducts that line the breast. This procedure could identify small lesions. As with the other technologies mentioned, this technique is not suitable for screening and should be used only as an adjunct to mammography.[39]

These new imaging techniques pose no radiation risk and do not require compression of the breast. None, however, is appropriate for mass screening; mammography is still the most effective mass screening technology presently available.

## LOW-TECH OPTIONS

While the advances in sophisticated imaging devices have done much to increase the accuracy and precision of breast cancer diagnosis, there is clearly a role for low-tech screening. The above-described devices are expensive and not appropriate for every woman, nor are they designed as first-line screening devices. Two of the most important nontechnical mechanisms for detecting abnormalities in the breast are breast self-exam (BSE) and clinical breast exam (CBE).

### Breast Self-Exam

Not every cancer is found by mammography, and not every woman undergoes routine mammogram screening; therefore, every woman should be taught how to examine her own breasts. BSEs should be done several days after menstruation ends, a time when the breasts are less likely to be swollen and tender.

Learning how to examine one's breasts and becoming familiar with the lumps and bumps helps an individual to detect a change in the texture of her breasts and could provide some reassurance that lumpy areas are normal. For example, the upper and outer areas around the armpit tend to be more lumpy than other parts of the breast. It is important to stress that most breast lumps are not cancer. Many lumps are fluid-filled cysts that can be left alone or can be drained. Fibrous breasts will feel lumpy, but are usually normal. The average-size lump found by regularly checking one's breasts are 2.1 cm compared to 1.1 cm to 1.5 cm found with mammography. The average-size lump found accidentally is 3.5 cm.

By performing a self-exam regularly, something that stands out as being different from the last time can be examined by a professional. Some women keep a journal noting lumps or irregularities. Changes in the texture and size (thickening or swelling) and discharge from the nipple or puckering/dimpling around the nipple are signs that something is not right. Any breast change from the normal may be a cause for concern. It is important to check all areas of the breast: the armpit to the collarbone, the breast itself, and the nipple area. Looking in a mirror helps visualize changes in shape, size, or skin texture. The self-exam can be done standing in the shower or lying down with a pillow under the shoulder. Feeling for lumps should be done in a circular manner using three fingers (not the tips of the fingers, the pads of the finger). Light, medium, and deep pressure should be applied. The right hand should be used to examine the left breast and the left hand should be used to examine the right breast.

## Clinical Breast Exam

A doctor or other trained health professional is qualified to perform a CBE. The exam includes an inspection of the breasts as well as palpation of the breast and chest area, including the lymph nodes above and below the collarbone and under each arm. Special attention is given to the shape and texture of the breasts, the location of any lumps, and the area around the armpits. It is often helpful if the CBE is scheduled within the same month as the mammogram since a CBE can alert the physician to unusual lumps that should be investigated further by mammography.

Clinical and self-breast exams are not substitutes for mammography. Mammography can often detect very small cancers two years before they can be discovered by physical exam. The sensitivity of CBE ranges from 48 to 69 percent whereas for mammography it is 75 to 90 percent. The specificity of the CBE is 85 to 99 percent.[40] However, CBE cannot differentiate malignant from benign palpable lesions, therefore, a further workup is required. Determining whether a lump is just a lump or whether it is more serious is the most difficult part of the CBE.

## SUMMARY

Breast cancer screening and mammography are synonymous in the public's mind. Although it has its limitations, mammography remains the most cost-efficient, safe, and cost-effective means of mass screening for breast cancer. While research is under way to test and assess a variety of procedures and techniques that one day may prove helpful in the diagnosis of early breast cancer, none of the procedures or techniques described in this chapter is as cost efficient for mass screening as mammography. The newer, sophisticated technologies are neither cost effective nor viable as a replacement for mammography at this time. However, they can be used as adjuncts to mammography in diagnosis and screening of suspicious lesions and can do so often without invasive (i.e., surgical) procedures. BSE and CBE, the low-tech options, should not be ignored as they have been shown to identify suspicious lumps that proved to be malignant.

It is important to understand that radiologists' accuracy of interpreting mammograms will vary. Those who read more mammograms have better accuracy than those who read fewer films. Clearly, the number of years of experience reading mammograms will affect accuracy as well. Aside from experience, other factors also influence radiologists' mammogram interpretation accuracy. The fear of a malpractice suit may subconsciously (or consciously) prompt a radiologist to overinterpret a mammogram, to be more cautious in his or her interpretation.

Clinical characteristics of the woman, too, will influence accuracy. Women who are taking HRT, for example, tend to have more dense breasts, which could reduce mammogram accuracy. Accuracy is more likely if menstruating women have a mammogram during the first or second week of the cycle when the breast tissue is less dense. Going to the same facility where previous films are stored could help accuracy because the radiologist could compare prior films to the current one. Or, if one is going to a different facility/office, obtaining a copy of prior films taken elsewhere and bringing it to where the mammogram will be performed would also help the radiologist in making comparisons.

Because no single imaging device can accurately detect all types of breast abnormalities in different types of breast tissue (dense and fatty breasts, breasts with implants, breasts with significant scarring), breast cancer screening should not necessarily be limited to one modality. Multiple imaging techniques are appropriate to detect and diagnose cancer in those individuals who have a suspicious mammogram. In some instances, however, these highly sophisticated imaging tests might detect more tumors but might also produce too many false alarms. The sensitivity and specificity of these tests need to be assessed. The costs of the tests, too, have to be taken into account. A mammogram costs a few hundred dollars, but a MRI costs thousands. The other tests discussed in this chapter are equally expensive. Clearly, the more sophisticated devices are not appropriate for mass screening at this time, but they are useful for high-risk women and for women who have abnormal mammograms.

## CHAPTER 6

# What Does the Research Show?

Preventing disease requires an understanding of the etiology, cause, and risk factors of the disease. Once causal and risk factors are identified, efforts can be mobilized to design programs to reduce the incidence of new disease or to eliminate the disease altogether. Since epidemiology looks at disease in population groups, not individuals per se, it cannot reliably answer the question: Why did this patient get this disease at this time? Epidemiology draws a larger picture and identifies risk factors that groups of individuals might have. While epidemiological studies are designed to identify risk factors, it does not mean that every identified risk factor will be present in every diseased individual. There is a natural biological variability among individuals. Not every smoker will get lung cancer, for example, even though smoking is a known risk factor for that disease.

Studies are conducted for a variety of reasons: to quantify disease risk or to show that one treatment or drug is better than another; to confirm or to refute preliminary clinical impressions regarding the origins of diseases. Ascertaining the meaning and strength of the relationship relies on statistical analyses. Whether a statistical association is found or not, several questions can and should be asked: Are the findings believable? Are there factors in the study design or in the study sample that could have biased the results? Are there potentially other factors that could explain the findings? How strong is the statistical association? In order to intelligently answer such questions, an understanding of the types of study design as well as the methodological problems inherent in any study is fundamentally important.

To a very large extent, the design of a study affects the quality of the data. Errors can and do arise in the process of designing and conducting a study. Cause and effect relationships and statistical associations can be misrepresented or misinterpreted if the study is designed poorly. Valid conclusions can be compromised. An analysis is only as good as the data on which it rests. Decisions made on the basis of faulty research gain no benefit and may be harmful.

## STUDY DESIGNS

Researchers design studies in different ways in order to draw conclusions about diseases and treatments. Different types of studies are appropriate for studying different kinds of questions. Logically, the appropriateness of the study design to the research question needs to be assessed. If one is looking to test a specific hypothesis, there are specific study designs that one would use. There are also specific types of study designs that one would use if looking to first decide on a hypothesis or hypotheses. There is a hierarchy in study design, which means that some studies produce more statistically certain findings than others. That is not to say that the study designs at the bottom of the hierarchy are not worthwhile or meaningless; rather, they add information but have methodological issues that make them not as "strong" as those study designs at the top of the hierarchy. There are essentially two major types of studies designs: observational and experimental.

Unlike experimental studies, observational studies do not introduce an intervention; there is no attempt to manipulate who is exposed to a factor and who is not. Individuals are observed over a specified time period. These studies are useful for hypothesis generation as well as for hypothesis testing in the search for the determinants of disease or for risk factors. Causal associations can be demonstrated statistically in two specific types of descriptive studies, the case control and the cohort studies. There are different types of observation studies ranging in hierarchy from more simple to more complex:

Case reports or case series studies focus on one single patient (case report) or a few patients. An interesting disease or diagnosis is reported, but no formal research study is conducted. For example, a report on the observation of systemic sclerosis among a small number of women with silicone gel breast implants could be presented as a case report or case series. Further research including a larger sample of women with breast implants would be needed to investigate scientifically the extent of the problem, the cause(s) of the disease, or means of treatment. Case report studies are the least valuable in terms of understanding disease etiology and disease causality.

*Cross-sectional studies* look at patterns of disease among a population at a specific point in time. They cannot link exposure with disease, but do provide a snapshot of what is happening at a particular point in time. They are useful to generate hypotheses, but do not test hypotheses. They also are useful to determine prevalence of a disease and to measure health status (e.g., how many people have diabetes at one point in time). National health surveys represent cross-sectional studies. While ranked higher than case reports, cross-sectional studies cannot determine causality.

*Case-control studies* test hypotheses in an effort to understand the etiology of a disease and possible risk factors for the disease. Individuals are studied for the specific purpose of determining whether or not the risk of disease is different among those exposed to a factor and those who are not. Case-control studies are retrospective because the data are collected on past events or experiences. The cases consist of individuals who have the disease of interest at the time of the study. The controls are disease free but are similar demographically and medically to the cases. The control group must have similar characteristics to the cases otherwise one runs the risk of compromising the study's validity. Controls should be matched on factors such as age, sex, geographic area to ensure comparability on key variables that could, themselves, explain some of the differences between the two groups.

These studies are designed primarily to assess the association between disease occurrence and a past exposure suspected of causing the disease. To determine whether an association between a disease and an exposure exists, one has to determine whether there is an excess risk of the disease in those who have been exposed to the agent or factor compared to those who have not been exposed. For example, in a study looking at breast cancer and HRT, the cases would be those with diagnosed breast cancer and the controls would be disease free. Comparison of use of HRT in both groups would be made. Calculation of the strength of association between exposure (HRT) and disease (breast cancer) is made, comparing the cases to the controls.

Case-control studies are very difficult to do well. Problems of bias, inappropriate selection of controls, reliance on historical data, data that are lost over time, patients' ability to recall or remember events surrounding exposure, and the like—individually and collectively—can serve to weaken the findings of a study.

*Cohort studies* follow individuals forward over time to assess who may or may not have been exposed to a factor thought to contribute to the development of disease and to see who develops disease and who does not. Whereas in a case-control study we know who has the disease and who does not, in a cohort study we sample a group of individuals who had the opportunity to be exposed to the factor of interest to see who develops the disease over time. For example, a cohort of women whose mothers had breast cancer and a group of similar women whose mothers did not have breast cancer are followed over time. The development of breast cancer in both groups is compared to assess the risk of disease associated with family history.

Cohort studies provide stronger evidence of causality than retrospective case-control studies. While these studies are less subject to bias and errors of recall, there are disadvantages such as the need for a large number of people to include in the study and the problem of individuals lost to follow-up. These studies are expensive to conduct, but they do provide a good description of disease progression and effects of exposure.

The gold standard for assessing causality is the *randomized clinical trial (RCT)*. Clinical trials are prospective, experimental studies that are much more rigorous than the case-control or cohort studies because individuals are assigned to receive and intervention or not. Analysis of the data assesses the effectiveness of the intervention (i.e., a drug or procedure). Trials should be designed to test one specific hypothesis or only a few hypotheses at a time. Rigorous procedures (protocols) are established in RCTs before individuals are admitted to the study. Once deemed eligible, an individual is randomly assigned to the experimental or the control group. The groups must be as similar to each other as possible so that differences in outcome can be attributed to the effect of the intervention. Randomization helps equalize the groups.

In a double-blind RCT, for example, neither the physician nor the patient knows who is getting the experimental treatment and who is not. This technique helps minimize bias; each individual is treated the same without prejudice since the treating physician would not know who is getting the intervention. For example, a study designed to look at the effect of tamoxifen among breast cancer patients would first list an inclusion and exclusion protocol (who is eligible to be in the study and who is not). Those who met the inclusion criteria would be randomized to receive the treatment or the placebo. Each woman would be given an identical looking pill (either the real drug or a placebo). Neither the physician nor the patient would know whether the real drug was being given or not. The group would be followed for a specified period of time during which clinical and nonclinical data would be collected. At the end of the trial, it would be revealed which group received tamoxifen and which received the placebo, and the results would be analyzed statistically to assess differences between the groups.

There are several types of clinical trials. Phase I and Phase II trials involve a very small number of people, and the purpose is to learn how to administer a drug safely and determine patients' responses to the drug. Patients are monitored closely for side effects. If the objective of the drug is to treat breast cancer, for example, individuals are monitored to see if their tumor shrinks during treatment. If at least one-fifth of the participants respond to the treatment, the drug is considered successful. If enough patients respond positively to the drug, a Phase III trial can be designed.

Phase III trials involve a large number of people and the FDA is involved in setting the standards and expectations for the trial. In these trials, individuals are randomly assigned to treatment or placebo group and outcomes measured. Participants are closely monitored for side effects. In some other trials, a standard treatment or drug is compared to a new treatment or new drug. The methodology is the same as described above. After clinical trials are completed, the findings should provide evidence of the treatment or drug's effectiveness and if the treatment or drug is safe (benefits outweigh the risks).

While the results of clinical trials help clinicians determine the superiority or inferiority of a specific treatment, drug, or therapy, it is very important for the clinician to be aware of the characteristics of the study population. How similar are the demographic and clinical characteristics of a clinician's patient to those in the RCT? If the RCT focused on white males, would the results be applicable to white females, or to African American males or females? Selection of study characteristics may limit the ability to generalize the findings to other patient population groups. Moreover, were the study participants hospitalized patients or ambulatory patients? Hospitalized patients might be sicker than the general population; therefore, their generalizability might be limited.

RCTs are really the best way to determine conclusively whether a new or modified treatment regimen is more effective than the existing one. Despite the importance of clinical trials, low enrollment rates in breast cancer trials have hampered therapeutic advancement in the field. Less than half of patients eligible for a trial choose to enroll. Those who do enroll in a trial sometimes have an unacceptably low level of understanding of the purpose of the trial, the risks, and the benefits.

In some instances, a physician may be reluctant to encourage his or her patients to join clinical trials. Physicians are concerned that patients will equate an attempt to enroll them in a clinical trial with an attempt to "experiment" on them. Or, patients may want to be guaranteed that they will receive the drug and not the placebo. Trials do not work that way. The purpose is to assess which therapy or drug is better than either existing therapy or drugs or placebo.

It is understandable that a patient could be uncomfortable with allowing the treatment to be assigned at random. What this patient may not understand, however, is that it could be that the placebo treatment is the current gold standard therapy against which the new therapy is being compared. Furthermore, a patient may not fully understand that clinical trials are required to have detailed inclusion and exclusion criteria designed to guarantee that the intervention being studied is appropriate for the patient. This is one of the central tenets of the modern-day clinical trial.

How does one "get into" a clinical trial? There are numerous commercial clinical trial sites on the Internet, but these are not subject to monitoring by institutional review boards (panels that examine ethical issues of a trial) unlike most trials conducted at academic medical centers, for example. Most pharmaceutical companies fund clinical trials and contract with academic medical centers to administer and analyze the data. Physicians can recruit patients for trials, and patients can ask their physician for trial options. Regardless of the source of the trial's funding, there is no guarantee that potential candidates will be accepted into the trial. Every trial has inclusion criteria and exclusion criteria.

Ultimately, the responsibility for informing the patient of the benefits of participating in clinical trials for both herself/himself and for society rests on the physician. This is primarily an exercise in effective communication. The physician must have the ability to introduce and sufficiently explain the clinical trial so as to avoid alienating the patient and being perceived as a researcher more than a caregiver.

Any individual who is considering participating in a clinical trial should find out as much information as possible about the nature and scope of the trial as well as the potential risks and benefits of the treatment. There are a number of online resources that one could consult (see end of chapter).

## CONSIDERATIONS OF STUDY DESIGN FLAWS

Regardless of the study design, there are certain factors that must be taken into account in order for the study findings to be considered meaningful. Control of sources of bias must be incorporated into the study design. That is, bias can occur if the selection of study patients is faulty, if the assignment of patients to treatment groups is unequal, or if the method of measuring outcomes or study endpoints is incorrect. Bias will cause the study results to mask the true values and thus compromise the study's validity and usefulness. Confounding, too, must be considered in study design. For example, smoking may be a confounding variable in a study investigating the relationship between coffee and heart disease because coffee drinkers are also smokers. Is it the coffee drinking that explains the development of heart disease or the smoking? It is important to take into account bias and confounding when designing a study as well as when analyzing the data. Wrong or misleading inferences from the study's findings could be made if these factors are not taken into account.

The size and duration of the study is important to consider. There should be enough people in the study to have statistical meaning. If study findings are based on a small sample of people, there will be less statistical relevance and less generalizabilty. If the study is conducted for a short period of time, statistically significant results may not be evident. For example, a six-month study looking at the effect of a specific medication to reduce blood pressure to prevent heart attack may need more time for the endpoint (heart attack) to occur. How likely an event being studied will occur and in what length of time should dictate the breadth and scope of the study design.

## WHAT DOES IT ALL MEAN?

While some studies produce more certain findings than others, there are advantages and disadvantages as well as constraints (financial, ethical, methodological) to any study design. The type of study design depends on the questions posed. In the hierarchy of study designs, RCTs are the most rigorous approach to compare the benefits of alternative treatments, while the case-control and cohort studies can calculate risk of an exposure or factor to disease. However, regardless of the study design, independent confirmation by other studies investigating the same issue is imperative. Rarely does one study bring about a major change in disease treatment or prevention; in almost all cases, replication of study findings is important before medical practice is changed. With this in mind, what do the studies on effectiveness of mammography show?

## WHAT DO THE STUDIES SHOW?

The value of screening mammography has been examined in scores of case-control studies and randomized clinical trials conducted over the past decades. The studies were designed to compare breast cancer mortality between those who received mammogram screening and those who did not. The benefit derived from mammography screening would be in the early detection of breast carcinomas at an early and more treatable stage, resulting in a reduction in mortality. Would mammography make a difference in saving lives was the question that needed to be answered.

The large-scale mammography studies conducted in the United States, Canada, and Europe differed in study design, eligibility considerations, study population characteristics, interventions (screening protocols differed), study outcomes, duration of follow-up over time, and analysis of outcomes. These design differences make it very hard to compare and contrast findings and equally difficult to make recommendations about who should be screened and how often. Nonetheless, the degree to which mammography reduces mortality is a central and important aspect of the debate.

Many of the major studies demonstrated reductions in breast cancer mortality, which led to the general acceptance of mammography as an important screening tool. However, all of the studies were conducted on healthy women, the overwhelming majority of whom would not develop breast cancer. Of those who developed breast cancer, only a minority would die from it. Point in fact: Every study showed relatively small numbers of breast cancer deaths in comparison to the large number of individuals included in the study.

The trials included almost 500,000, women and each study tried to quantify the benefits of mammogram screening. For better or for worse, the findings from each of the trials contributed to the ongoing debate about mammography's effectiveness on women of different ages. Many were criticized for methodological flaws, some more serious than others. Proponents and critics alike found a basis to support their position, each relying on the same data but drawing different conclusions. The following briefly summarizes the key components of eight of the major large-scale trials.

*The Health Insurance Plan (HIP) Study,* initiated in New York in 1963, was the first large-scale randomized clinical mammography trial.[1] Approximately 60,000 women aged forty to sixty-four were matched on key factors and randomized to have mammograms and clinical breast exams or not. (The actual number of women in the trial is unclear, as it has been reported differently in publications). The follow-up duration was as long as eighteen years. Although randomization should have produced equal distribution of women in the two groups, there were significant imbalances in the distribution of women with prior breast lumps, menopause, and education. Furthermore, researchers decided that they did not want to include women who already had breast cancer, and these women were dropped from the study after they were randomized. About 1,100 women were dropped—800 from the mammography group and 300 from the control group. Hence, more women with preexisting breast cancer were excluded from the screening group than from the control group. This difference introduced bias in favor of the screening group. These biases are important to consider when evaluating the implications of the findings. The debate as to whether this decision biased the study's conclusions that mammography led to a lower breast cancer death rate continues to this day.

Study findings published in 1971 showed that mammography reduced breast cancer deaths by 30 percent. That is, the breast cancer death rate was 30 percent higher in women who did not have mammograms. Of the approximately 31,000 who were not screened, 124 died of breast cancer compared with 81 of the approximately 31,000 who were screened by mammography. Despite the serious questions raised about the randomization process, the researchers concluded that women should be encouraged to have mammograms to screen for breast cancer. There was no recommendation made based on the age of the woman.

From 1977 to 1983, four randomized trials were initiated in Europe to investigate the potential benefits of mammogram screening. *The Malmo, Sweden, trial* began in 1976 and lasted twelve years.[2] Unlike the HIP study, randomization of approximately 42,000 women aged forty-five to sixty-nine was done by birth-year cohort (cluster randomization—those on the first half of the lists were invited for screening). There were 21,000 women in the screening group and 21,200 in the control group, and the randomization produced similar groups. Women with preexisting breast cancer were excluded from the screening group, but not the control group. Findings showed that more breast cancer deaths occurred in the screened population than in the controls until year seven, after which the trend reversed. Among women aged forty-five to fifty-five at the beginning of the study, this persisted until year ten. The Malmo Study is viewed as being of acceptable quality; any flaws in study design are considered minimal and do not bias the findings. The study showed that mammography screening lowered breast cancer mortality.

*The Edinburgh trial* was initiated in 1976 and followed women between the ages of forty-five and sixty-four for up to ten years.[3] Approximately 23,200 women were in the screened group and 21,900 in the control group. Cluster randomization was based on physician practices. Criticism of this trial focused on the method of randomization. The groups differed substantially at baseline; indeed, the randomization method was deemed grossly inadequate, even for a cluster analysis. The problem focused on socioeconomic differences between study and control groups, as only 26 percent of the women in the control group were in the highest socioeconomic group whereas 53 percent of those in the screened group were. Differences in SES among practices were not recognized until after the study ended. Furthermore, there were more women with preexisting breast cancer who were excluded from the screened group than from the control group. Because of these factors, this trial is considered flawed.

The first *Canadian National Breast Screening Study* was initiated in 1980. This individually randomized trial was the only trial specifically designed to study women aged forty to forty-nine at study entry and to evaluate the efficacy of annual mammography, breast physical examination, and instruction on BSE in reducing breast cancer mortality.[4] That is, breast cancer mortality would be compared between (1) women who received screening with annual mammography, BSE, and instruction on BSE on four or five occasions, and (2) women who received community care after a single breast physical examination and instruction on BSE. Of the 50,430 volunteers, approximately 25,000 women aged were randomized to the screened group, and 25,000 women were randomized to the control group (usual community care with annual follow-up). Before randomization, each woman received an initial breast physical examination and instruction on BSE. The groups were similar at baseline.

After eleven to sixteen years of follow-up, the women receiving mammography and breast examinations did not have reduced breast cancer mortality compared to those women who received usual community care (no screening by mammography). The researchers concluded that based on their findings, there was no statistical benefit of mammography in women under age fifty.

The second Canadian National Breast Screening Study, conducted in 1980, focused on women aged fifty to fifty-nine.[5] In this trial, 39,405 women in that age group were randomly assigned to receive mammography plus breast physical examination or physical examination only. Almost 20,000 women were in the screened group, and almost 20,000 were in the control group. The average follow-up was thirteen years (ranging from eleven to sixteen years). This trial found that in women between the ages of fifty and fifty-nine, the addition of annual mammography screening to physical examination had apparently no impact on breast cancer mortality; that is, it was not beneficial in reducing breast cancer mortality. The researchers state, however, that their findings do not negate the reported benefit from mammography screening when compared with no screening at all.

*The Stockholm, Sweden, trial* of 1981 focused on women aged forty to sixty-four.[6] Women with preexisting breast cancer were excluded from the screened group but not the control group. Randomization was based on date of birth, with women born on days eleven through twenty of any month comprising the control group. There is substantial discrepancy of the actual number of women in each group; the number of women in the screened group declined by 2,000 individuals and rose 1,000 in the control group from the beginning of the study to the final report. The researchers could not explain this inconsistency, but it certainly appears that the randomization method may have been inadequate. Statistics indicate that in this study the mammogram was not protective.

In the *Gothenburg, Sweden, trial* initiated in 1982, women between the ages of forty and fifty-nine were followed for eleven years.[7] Randomization was partly by day-of-birth cluster and partly individual. Analysis showed that women were significantly younger in the screened group compared to the control group. Women with preexisting breast cancer were excluded from the screened group but not the control group. Results of the forty to forty-nine cohort oddly found that the control group had a higher cancer incidence than the screened group, and there were higher than expected cancer incidence in both groups.

Two other Swedish trails, *Kopparberg* and *Ostergotland* were conducted in the 1980s as well.[8] Cluster randomization was used based on dividing the population in these counties into nineteen blocks, which were further divided into two or three groups on unspecified criteria. The groups were then randomized. Assessment of these studies concluded that the women in the screened group in both studies were older than the control group, skewing the distribution and raising questions about the validity of the randomization process. Furthermore, the actual number of women randomized is not clear as different numbers were reported at different times.

In addition to the clinical trials, many population-based studies looked at mammography screening and breast cancer outcomes. The *Breast Cancer Detection Demonstration Project (BCDDP)* was a national mammography screening program conducted from 1973 to 1981 at twenty-nine U.S. centers.[9] This study was a prospective, cohort study in which there was no randomization. Approximately 283,000 women were followed over many years, and long-term follow-up found very high survival rates in younger as well as older women. Among a cohort of 4,240 women with a histologically confirmed diagnosis of breast cancer, the five-, eight-, and ten-year survival rates were over 80 percent. This study looked carefully at the value of screening women before age fifty. Comparisons of breast cancers detected and survival rates between those younger than age fifty to those in their fifties showed that screening was as effective in the younger women as in the older women. It seems that there were substantial gains in survival primarily because a high proportion of cancers were being diagnosed and treated at early stages.

Another study looking at the potential benefits of mammography screening in two Swedish counties found that regular mammogram screening resulted in a 63 percent reduction in breast cancer deaths among women who underwent screening.[10] In this study, data on the death rate in women who actually used screening was compared to those who were not screened. Records were examined for almost 7,000 women who developed breast cancer and for almost 2,000 women who died of breast cancer over a twenty-nine-year period. The researchers analyzed only those cancers and deaths within the three time periods (1968–1977, 1978–1987, and 1988–1996). The mortality from incident breast cancer, diagnosed in women between forty and sixty-nine years of age who were screened during the period 1988–1996, declined by 63 percent compared with breast cancer mortality during the time period 1968–1977 when no screening was available. They concluded that screening substantially reduced breast cancer mortality in the two counties in Sweden. It must be stated, however, that mammography screening in the two counties had been in existence for many years and the compliance rate was very high (over 85 percent). Whether other countries could reproduce these findings needs to be determined. The randomized clinical trials discussed earlier did not show such robust benefits of screening with regard to reducing mortality.

## DOES SCREENING "WORK"?

Based on years of following tens of thousands of women and accumulating mounds of data, what conclusions can be drawn regarding the affect of mammography screening on breast cancer mortality? To what extent are lives extended because of early breast cancer detection? To what extent does mammography screening improve overall survival?

Although few of the large-scale trials were methodologically perfect, most showed varying reductions in breast cancer mortality. Only the Canadian trial failed to find such a benefit, regardless of age of the woman; no differences in survival rates between women who were screened by physical exam compared to women who were screened by physical exam and mammography were found.[11] This particular study has been criticized the most, perhaps because it was the one to show the most negative results. The other large-scale trials generally showed that screening is beneficial and that reduced mortality from breast cancer among women aged fifty and older, in particular, is evident. As such, there was general agreement that screening mammography for women aged fifty to sixty-nine is beneficial, in spite of the weak findings and methodological issues just delineated.

Why did some studies show a benefit and these failed to do so? Drawing definitive conclusions from the data is complicated by the difficulties in designing population-screening trials. All of the trials had limitations and methodological flaws, some being more serious than others. The randomization process in most of the trials failed to create similar groups, making an unbiased assessment difficult. The actual number of women in each group could not be determined in several of the studies (Stockholm, Kopparberg, Ostergotland, and the HIP study), raising questions as to what effect this had on the study findings. Differences in training of radiologists and differences in mammography techniques have been raised as possible sources of bias; it is well known that mammography performance is dependent on the expertise of the radiologist. Also, the issue of variable age at entry into the trials (forty to forty-nine versus over age fifty) may contribute to differences in when mammographic screening was begun.

While the BCDDP study (not a randomized trial) found benefits of screening younger (under age fifty) as well as older women (over age fifty), no other study's findings were strong enough to extend this recommendation to women younger than age fifty. So, what should be recommended to these younger women? Women in their forties have a lower cancer incidence compared to women older than age fifty, but the cancers in the younger women tend to be more aggressive. Also, mammogram interpretations of premenopausal, dense breast tissue are notoriously difficult. Would the potential benefit of early mammogram screening be evident among women younger than age fifty? The data from the large-scale trials could not answer that question.

## WHAT'S NEXT?

To some, the problems of the trials raised questions about the reliability of the findings, leading some to question screening effectiveness. A few even advocated that mammograms not be performed routinely because they do not reduce breast cancer mortality. Meanwhile, scores of governmental and professional associations had strongly endorsed (and continue to do so) the annual mammogram as a means of early detection and treatment for breast cancer.

In 1990, for example, Congress passed the Breast and Cervical Cancer Mortality Prevention Act of 1990, which authorized the Centers for Disease Control and Prevention to provide breast and cervical cancer screening services to older women, women with low incomes, and underserved women of racial and ethnic minority groups. The National

Breast and Cervical Cancer Early Detection Program (NBCCEDP) provided free mammograms to those who could not afford routine breast cancer screening. During its first decade, the program provided nearly 1.2 million mammogram screening tests and 1.3 million Pap tests from which 8,000 breast and cervical cancers were detected and diagnosed.

In October 2000, commemorating Breast Cancer Awareness Month, the Secretary of Health and Human Services reiterated the government's commitment to breast cancer detection and screening. Government support not withstanding, some researchers had expressed doubts about the effectiveness of mammography. This debate had been limited to the professional journals, but soon spilled out to the lay press and naturally created quite a controversy. Epidemiologists and biostatisticians needed to clarify the issue, and women, confused by this new wrinkle, were wondering whether or not they should have annual or biannual mammograms. And then things became truly complicated when Danish researchers, after reassessing the data, announced that screening mammography does not confer survival benefit for breast cancer, regardless of age.

## WEB SITES FOR ONLINE CLINICAL TRIAL LISTINGS (NOT COMPREHENSIVE)

www.clinicaltrials.gov This National Institutes of Health site features a searchable database and detailed trial descriptions.

www.cancer.gov/clinicaltrials This National Cancer Institute site features an extensively searchable database and trial descriptions are available.

www.clinicaltrials.cancer.org This American Cancer Society site features a searchable database as well as descriptions of trials available.

www.centerwatch.com This site provides minimal descriptions but one can sign up for more information.

www.clinicaltrials.com This site is hosted by Pharmaceutical Research Plus, Inc.

www.veritasmedicine.com This site is hosted by a private corporation and has a searchable database with a simplified search results.

www.imaginis.com/breasthealth/bc This site enables individuals to learn more about FDA-approved drugs used to treat breast cancer.

www.fda.gov/cder This site provides information on the FDA's approval and regulatory processes—Center for Drug Evaluation and Research (CDER).

www.cancernet.nci.nih.gov Government-funded studies such as those at the National Cancer Institute are posted on this site.

## CHAPTER 7

# Science, Politics, and Mammograms

Consider a woman in her mid-forties with an average risk of breast cancer. Should she have annual mammogram screenings? Would the benefits from mammography justify potential "harm," such as a false positive result, that would necessitate additional diagnostic workup? Certainly, detecting breast cancer at an early stage is important and potentially beneficial, but this woman has no way of knowing whether in the next decade she will be one of the majority who does not get breast cancer or one of the few who will. The data seem to indicate that regular screening confers only a small benefit for women in their forties who do not have an increased risk for breast cancer, such as a primary relative who has had breast cancer. But, what may be a marginal benefit epidemiologically may not be perceived as such by an individual.

Each woman is unique, and her risk of breast cancer will vary by age, ethnicity, family history, genetics, and biology, among other factors. The annual risk of a sixty-year-old woman being diagnosed with breast cancer is greater than that of a forty-year-old woman, and the older woman has a greater likelihood of dying from the disease. Mammogram screening recommendations logically need to reflect these differences. Furthermore, the issue of optimal intervals between screening mammograms, while not clear, has great implications. Cancers that arise between screening exams (interval cancers) have characteristics of rapid growth and are frequently of advanced stage. So, who should be screened? At what age? How frequently?

There are differences of opinion regarding at what age to initiate screening, how frequently screening should be done, and for whom. The long-term effect of mammogram screening, in general, and its effect on survival, in particular, are subject to differences of opinion. Although those debating the issue are relying on the same data, their conclusions are at odds. If the experts cannot agree, what is the layperson supposed to believe?

## MAMMOGRAPHY DILEMMA

Decisions about whether to offer mass screening are difficult and complex, and involve an assessment of the potential benefits of screening against the potential harms. Clearly, if the harms outweigh the benefits, screening should not be offered. If early detection does not result in better outcomes, there is no point in offering screening. If there is evidence that screening results in better outcomes but only for a small number of people, the harms of screening a large number of people need to be assessed. With mammography screening, there is a potentially large benefit for a small number of individuals, and a potentially small amount of harm for a much larger number. Because screening involves primarily healthy women, the potential benefits and harms of the screening mechanism must be assessed, and the limitations of the screening technology be acknowledged.[1] Unfortunately, there is no clear cutoff for deciding when the benefits outweigh the harms.

Rational decision making, be it for the individual or for population groups, should be based on sound data, but if there are disagreements in the interpretation of the statistics, the process becomes much more complicated. If the data on which policy recommendations are made are suspect or flawed, decision making will be compromised. As discussed earlier, poor randomization, small sample size, and questionable generalizability of the study population can compromise the validity of any study. These issues are central to the mammogram controversy.

The benefit of mammogram screening focuses on detecting breast cancer at an early stage so that treatment can begin with the hope of extending lives. Saving lives, after all, is the basic premise of early disease detection. Screening for cancers of the breast, colon, cervix, and prostate, for example, is advocated because early intervention and treatment can improve survival and hopefully improve quality of life for cancer survivors. As was explained in an earlier chapter, to be effective, any screening test should have a high sensitivity and specificity, and early detection should not only reduce the rate of death, but also the number of false positive tests should be relatively low.

It also is important to note that screening does not reduce the risk for being *diagnosed* with breast cancer; it is meant to reduce the risk for *dying* of breast cancer. The literature is consistent in advocating early screening and detection for breast cancer even though screening mammography does not detect all tumors nor prevent all deaths from breast cancer. In all fairness, at this point in time, technology cannot detect all tumors, and the newer, more sophisticated technologies discussed earlier are not yet appropriate to serve as a replacement for X-ray film mammography. Digital mammography, ultrasound, and MRI are very good adjuncts to mammography in diagnosis and screening, for example, but they are not replacements for mammography.

There have been numerous case-control studies and randomized controlled trials, including nearly half a million women from four countries, that have compared breast cancer mortality of women who were screened to those who were not. There have been hundreds of opinion pieces and editorials commenting on the findings of these studies. Yes, the trials differed in population recruitment, method of randomization, and analysis of outcomes, and these differences in design and analysis methodology create problems in data comparison. The studies are conducted on healthy women, the overwhelming majority of whom will not develop cancer. Nevertheless, based on the trial results, there had been a general agreement that screening mammography for women aged fifty to sixty-nine is beneficial. There was no clear agreement regarding recommendations for younger women, although there may be a small benefit in favor of screened women in their forties, ten to twelve years after the initiation of screening.[2]

Of all the large trials, only one, the Canadian National Breast Screening Study, found that annual mammography screening had no appreciable impact on breast cancer mortality. It was the only study to show no beneficial effect of mammography, regardless of age. The researchers posited that if mammography does indeed make a difference, it would have been evident after seven years of follow-up. These results were not evident. The study's controversial findings were not widely accepted by the medical community, and most key organizations, including the ACS, did not accept the findings. What makes the Canadian study findings so different from that of other studies? Why was that study the only one to find no beneficial effect from mammography? Rather than delve further to try to answer these questions, most organizations and the medical community chose to ignore the findings and continued to advocate for mammography.

## THE CRUX OF THE CONTROVERSY

In January 2000, Danish researchers revisited the issue of breast cancer screening. Researchers at the Nordic Cochrane Center in Copenhagen critically looked at the individual trials to see if breast cancer mortality has decreased as a result of mammogram screening. The Nordic Cochrane Center is a highly respected group of researchers who use rigorous and well-developed methods for conducting systematic reviews. It was their opinion that all but two of the trials were so flawed in design that the results were unreliable. That is, these studies might have found benefits when in fact there were none, or they might have exaggerated what benefits there were.

The Danish researchers were highly critical of both the randomization methods used in the trials as well as the eligibility considerations.[3] Women, it seems, were more likely to be excluded as a result of a prior diagnosis of breast cancer if they were in the screened group. Since any breast cancer survivor has a greater chance of ultimately dying of breast cancer, this could certainly bias the conclusions. Further, in these trials, more women died of causes other than breast cancer than die of breast cancer, thus questioning the ability of the trials to detect reliably the impact of mammography on overall mortality. That is, knowledge of screening status may affect the judgment of cause of death, according to the researchers.

The degree to which mammography reduces mortality is an important issue in the debate. Cause of death likely differed among women who were screened compared to those who were not. The Danish researchers concluded that based on their review of the data, screening for breast cancer with mammography did not decrease breast cancer mortality, and therefore screening should not be recommended. They came to the dramatic conclusion that screening for breast cancer with mammography is unjustified (their term) because there is no reliable evidence that it reduces mortality.

The Danish researchers could find no statistical evidence that screening decreases breast cancer mortality, the main outcome measure in the screening trials. For every 1,000 women screened biannually for twelve years, one breast cancer death is avoided while the total number of deaths is increased by six. They also opined that the methodological quality of the screening trials was poor, making it difficult to base recommendations on the data. Clearly, this conclusion created a storm of debate and criticism.

When the Nordic Cochrane researchers submitted their review to the editors of the Breast Cancer Group of the Cochrane Collaboration based in Oxford, England, they found that their conclusions were unwelcome. The editors insisted on changes to the text, which would lend support to arguments in favor of screening and exclude data about the effects of screening on subsequent treatment. The Danish researchers refused to make the changes, and the *Lancet* decided to publish the findings as written, but also included a review of how the Cochrane Collaboration came to view the Danish researchers' work.[4]

In October 2001, the same researchers published a reassessment of their findings and again asserted that mammograms do not indicate any survival benefit for breast cancer. In fact, they concluded that the estimated mammography effect on all cause mortality is negligible.[5] This second review confirmed and strengthened their previous findings. Women who were screened tended to have more invasive tests done to follow up on inconclusive or suspicious mammograms. Yet, their death rates were no different from those who were not screened. This conclusion, directly challenging the traditional belief that mammograms saved lives, stunned the breast cancer research community and further fueled the debate.

The Danish critique of the data not only called into question the value of mammography for women younger than age fifty, it also threw into doubt the benefit of mammography for older women. While there always has been disagreement over many aspects of breast cancer screening, the dramatic pronouncement that mammograms do not save lives and, in fact, cause many women to undergo uncomfortable and costly follow-up procedures, had experts rushing to reevaluate the evidence. Those who were advocating mammogram screening for all women over forty prior to the Danish publication affirmed their belief in the value of screening. The flaws inherent in the studies that the Danish researchers discounted were not severe enough to discount the body of evidence, in their opinion. Those who had not put much stock in mammography used the Danish findings to bolster their viewpoint, which was (and perhaps may still be) that mammograms have drawbacks leading at times to excessive treatments for tumors that would not have threatened a woman's life but would entail expensive workup.

This strong anti-mammography screening stance created a furor. All recommendations regarding mammogram screening were based on data from the same trials that were included in the Danish reanalysis. As flawed as these studies may be, nonprofit organizations and the U.S. government agencies involved in setting screening recommendations felt that the benefits of screening far outweighed the negatives. Furthermore, the issue is an emotionally and politically charged one. Saying that mammogram screening does not work goes against deeply held beliefs.

Other researchers looking at the contribution of mammography screening to reductions in mortality have concluded that screening has made a difference. Data from the Regional Oncology Centres in Uppsala and Linkoping, Sweden, were used to compare deaths from breast cancer that was diagnosed in the twenty years before screening was introduced (1958–1977) with those from breast cancer diagnosed in the twenty years after the introduction of screening (1978–1997) in two Swedish counties.[6] The study population consisted of 210,000 women between the ages of twenty and sixty-nine years. The findings show that among women aged forty to sixty-nine who were screened, there was significantly lower breast cancer mortality compared to those diagnosed prescreening. Women in the same age range who were not exposed to screening had significantly higher breast cancer mortality. In the twenty to thirty-nine age group, there was no significant difference in breast cancer mortality in 1978 to 1997, compared with 1958 to 1977. The researchers concluded that mammography screening contributed to the substantial reductions in breast cancer mortality among women over age forty.

Other studies also have shown the benefits of mammography in younger as well as older women.[7] Gains in survival are perhaps a result of a high proportion of cancers being diagnosed and treated at more favorable stages as a result of early detection screening. Another benefit from screening is that it allows the patient a wider choice of treatment options. But, the Canadian National Breast Screening Study, the only one of the trials not to have found a benefit for mammography combined with physical breast exam compared with physical exam alone, continued to show that annual mammography for up to five years did not reduce breast cancer mortality.[8] And, the disagreements continue with proponents of mammography saying that screening has helped detect many more early tumors and that declines in later-stage cancers show that screening is beneficial. Mammography's strength is detecting tumors confined to the breast ducts. Critics dismiss this and say that the rates of later-stage cancers have not declined significantly since the use of mammography became widespread.

Many now feel that there is compelling evidence to show that mammography has benefits and that it is time to move on.[9] In an updated review of the Swedish randomized trials, researchers extended the follow-up and analyzed the age-specific and trial-specific effects on breast cancer mortality.[10] In a thoughtful analysis, the Swedish researchers concluded that there is a statistically significant reduction in breast cancer mortality, and the effect of breast screening on breast cancer mortality persists after long-term follow-up. In their opinion, the data affirm that screening mammography has a real but modest effect on mortality from breast cancer, although this effect varies with age. The reduction in breast cancer mortality is greatest among those sixty to sixty-nine at entry to the study, and there were statistically significant effects in the age groups fifty to fifty-nine, sixty to sixty-four, and sixty-five to sixty-nine. There was a small effect among those fifty to fifty-four. That is, the benefits of screening became statistically significant beginning at age fifty-five. Among fifty-five- to sixty-four-year-old women, deaths among those who were screened were reduced by 27 percent. Deaths were reduced 14 percent among those forty-five to fifty-four years old who were screened. Their conclusion, that the advantageous effect of breast screening on breast cancer mortality persists after long-term follow-up, directly challenges the Danish critique. The Swedish overview focuses on issues of randomization methodology and selection of participants, concerns raised by the Danish researchers. The Swedish study was, in many ways, methodologically a more robust meta-analysis.[11]

Meanwhile, as the debate continues, the National Cancer Institute continues to sponsor large trials to assess the potential of new breast cancer screening methods. Studies are presently under way to investigate the use of MRI for screening high-risk women. A trial comparing digital mammography to conventional film screen mammography is being conducted as well.

## SCREENING RECOMMENDATIONS?

Decisions about whether to offer mammogram screening in general, and to target specific cohorts in particular, are difficult and complex. There is a trade-off between the benefits of screening and its harms. While the debate about mammography's effectiveness continues, numerous nonprofit and public agencies continue to issue guidelines on mammography screening. Although each advocates mammography screening as the best way to detect early breast cancer, the guidelines differ on what age to begin screening (at age forty? fifty? or sixty?) and how frequently a woman should be screened (annually? biannually?).

For most cancer screening programs, there is only a relatively brief age range during which screening is worthwhile. Breast cancer is rare among very young women (younger than thirty-five, for example); only the very small number of individuals who potentially would benefit from screening would be outweighed by the much larger number of women who potentially could be harmed by regular screening (inconvenience, cost, false negative readings, etc.). As the incidence of breast cancer increases with age, the benefit of screening rises to the point where the harms might outweigh the benefits. That is, in the older woman (over age sixty-nine years, for example), the woman has fewer the years in which breast cancer can cause symptoms or death. At this age, there are competing factors such as heart disease or cardiovascular diseases that would result in death before the breast cancer would. Additionally, it is possible that a screening program for older women would detect more cancer, which would never be clinically important. In this situation, the benefits of screening is outweighed by the harms.

There is an age range during which mammogram screening is worthwhile: between the ages of fifty and sixty-nine years. In order to quantify when the trade-off between benefit and harm occurs (when the harms outweigh the benefits), the size of the mortality benefit from screening should be calculated as well as the potential harms of screening such as unnecessary workup for false positive results. It is not as easy as it sounds.

### The Younger Woman

The debate about the potential magnitude of the benefit of screening mammography for women in their forties has been ongoing for years.

Mammograms miss up to 25 percent of breast cancer in women in their forties compared to 10 percent for women in their fifties and older.[12] It is well accepted that mammograms of younger (premenopausal) women are more difficult to read. Among this cohort, there are more false positive readings, which entail further testing. The overwhelming majority of these cases end up not having cancer, but the discomfort, anxiety, and cost of undergoing tests must be factored in the equation. Additionally, there are more false negative readings among this cohort compared to women over age fifty. Complicating the picture is the fact that women in their early forties are biologically different from those in their late forties, and this has to be addressed as well.

There have been several meta-analyses on breast cancer screening among women between the ages of forty and forty-nine years. A major difficulty with interpreting the evidence from these analyses, however, is that the trials on which they are based either enrolled women between forty and forty-nine years or between forty-five and forty-nine years, but not women aged forty years. Hence, the question, "What is the incremental benefit of beginning screening at age forty rather than at age fifty?" is difficult to answer.

Basing decisions on data from the eight randomized clinical trials, a large demonstration project, case-control studies, and meta-analyses, the general consensus is that overall, the results are mixed, showing mortality reduction for the forty to forty-nine-year-old cohort, and, for the most part, the benefit of screening women in their forties can be attributable to screening that occurs after age fifty. Irwig and colleagues, in their review of the evidence about the value of mammography screening in forty- to forty-nine-year-old women, concluded that approximately 2,600 women in that age group would need to be screened to prevent one death from breast cancer thirteen years later.[13] Applying their model to a hypothetical cohort of 10,000 women who were offered screening every two years beginning at age forty, the expected benefit would be a saving of seven lives after thirteen years per 10,000 women invited to begin screening at age forty rather than at age fifty. Of these 10,000 women, 2,000 would have an abnormal mammogram and would be recalled for further assessment. The overwhelming majority of these women will not have breast cancer, Of the 2,000 with abnormal mammograms, 230 would require biopsies, of which 100 invasive cancers would be diagnosed and 21 women would be diagnosed with DCIS. The researchers conclude that the evidence to date shows a modest benefit of initiating screening from age forty rather than age fifty. Any benefit, however, would not be apparent until eight years after the commencement of screening. Furthermore, to be considered against these benefits are the increased rates of false positives and false negatives that will occur among this cohort.

The Irwig et al. model assumed that the forty- to forty-nine-year-old cohort was similar, but it could be argued that the benefit of screening would be greater in the older group (forty-five to forty-nine years) rather than in the younger group (under forty-five years). Age, however, is not the only risk factor for breast cancer. Those with a family history or identification of genetic mutations could gain a greater absolute benefit by screening in their forties. At this time there are no trials that tested whether screening would be beneficial for women at high risk of breast cancer. Intuitively, those who are at highest risk could expect to benefit more from screening. Screening women at increased risk of breast cancer from age forty should result in substantial benefits, and among these high-risk women, one would expect to prevent thirty deaths per 10,000 screened.

Because the detectable preclinical phase for breast cancer is shorter in younger women who develop breast cancer compared with that in women fifty years and older, a key issue that also is unresolved concerns an appropriate screening interval. Should there be annual screening or would a twenty-four-month screening interval be appropriate? The National Cancer Institute suggests that women in their forties have screenings every one to two years, depending on individual risk factors.[14] But, given the evidence, a universal recommendation for mammography for women in their forties is difficult to make. The most prudent course of action is for the individual to decide for herself, in consultation with her physician, whether and when to initiate mammogram screening. This decision should be based on the individual's risk factors for breast cancer and on her perceptions of risks and benefits of screening.

## The Older Woman

Breast cancer incidence and mortality rates increase with age. Almost half of new cases and nearly two-thirds of deaths from breast cancer occur in 13 percent of the female population sixty-five years and older. However, elderly women (over age sixty-five years) are less likely to have ever had a mammogram or to have had a recent mammogram in the past one to two years compared to younger women. Among those older women who are diagnosed with breast cancer, the disease is often at a later stage, making survival less likely and treatment choices more limited. Mammography can result in detection of earlier-stage breast cancer among older women, thus increasing the odds of increased survival, but there are risks inherent in advocating screening for all elderly women.[15]

The over sixty-five-year-old cohort is also heterogeneous. Women in their seventies, for example, are different from those between sixty-five and sixty-nine, and blanket recommendations should not be made for this reason. A recent systematic review designed to assess the benefits, harms, and costs of screening mammography in women age seventy and older found that the benefit of screening women seventy to seventy-nine years is 40 to 72 percent of that achieved in women age fifty to sixty-nine years and declines further with increasing age. The life expectancy benefit of screening mammography in older women diminishes with increasing age.[16] From an economic point of view, the central question is whether extending mammography screening beyond age sixty-nine, for example, represents value for money. Given the uncertainty, older women, in consultation with their physician, may want to decide for themselves whether or not to continue with mammography screening. Clearly, the choices women make will vary depending on how each values the possible benefits and risks.

Nevertheless, some organizations recommend screening mammography for women aged seventy and older despite the lack of clear evidence of benefit.[17] Although the data are limited, it is generally agreed that mammograms after age sixty-nine offer little benefit in gains in life expectancy.[18] Especially in this cohort, one needs to take into account the potential harms of mammography. Most of these women have comorbid conditions such as hypertension, heart disease, respiratory disease, and the like that will affect survival. Regardless of the stage at diagnosis of breast cancer, death from other causes is far more likely within three to five years. With reduced life expectancy to begin with, screening mammography will not likely affect overall mortality, but may indeed influence quality of life. That is, diagnostic workup of an abnormal mammogram must be taken into account, especially since the vast majority of these abnormal results would not represent cancer.

One could argue for targeting healthy older women rather than those with multiple health problems. For the healthy elderly, screening could be beneficial because early-stage disease detection could result in a reduction in breast cancer mortality. But a woman's preference for a possible small gain in life expectancy must be weighed against the potential harms of screening. For most women over age seventy, perhaps a CBE would be more appropriate. Overall, the evidence suggests that mammography offers the greatest potential benefit for women between fifty and sixty-nine years.

## SO, NOW WHAT?

The mammogram debate is far from settled. Researchers reviewing and analyzing the same data sets not only cannot agree at what age mammogram screening should be recommended, but also whether the benefits of mammogram screening outweigh the risks in the first place. Policymakers are equally confused and are perhaps reluctant to state publicly that mammography may not be valuable. The current debate makes it sound like an either-or decision, but the issue is more complex, more nuanced, than that. The magic cut-off of age fifty is arbitrary. How does one differentiate a forty-eight-year-old woman from a fifty-one-year-old woman? Weighing the costs against the benefits of mammography screening, as well as taking into account the psychological impact of false positive screening results, must be considered.

As was discussed, the body of evidence indicates that there is a benefit of mammography screening for women aged fifty to sixty-nine. After age sixty-nine, mammography screening offers minimal gains in life expectancy, and there are potential harms associated with screening that might outweigh the potential benefits. But, what should the woman between the ages of forty and forty-nine do? For this cohort, evidence that mammography reduces mortality from breast cancer is weak, and the absolute benefit of screening is smaller than it is for the older woman. Proponents and critics adhering to their position continue to enrich the debate. But, it is important to understand that they are basing their recommendations on population-based statistics derived from openly acknowledged studies with inherent methodological flaws. Although some have arrived at strikingly different conclusions about the benefits of mammography screening, the evidence can support guidelines that recommend breast cancer screening beginning at age forty or age fifty.

In truth, mammography's benefits have to be weighed against the potential risks and benefits for the individual woman as well as the associated costs (financial and emotional). Genetic and heredity risk factors that might predispose a woman to breast cancer must be taken into account. Individual risks, individual comfort levels, must be taken into account. While not every cancer will become deadly, physicians cannot predict which ones are dangerous and which ones are not. From the woman's perspective, how much harm is she willing to accept for an uncertain benefit?

The question of who should be screened for breast cancer, at what age, and how often is not simply an academic debate. There are factors other than the statistical results of a study that must be taken into account. As discussed earlier, ethnic differences, among other factors, need to be addressed. Despite overall lower incidence of disease when compared to white women, African American women have higher breast cancer mortality. While there have been significant improvements in mammography screening utilization, African American women and Hispanic women are still not receiving the full benefit. Strategies to increase mammography screening to ensure that minority women obtain the same benefits as white women need to be thought out. With early detection and with follow-up of abnormal mammograms, improved survival should be seen. Given that minority women, especially African American women, have poorer prognosis primarily because their breast cancers are detected at a later stage, serious consideration of initiating screening for those aged forty and older should be given.[19]

## WHAT DO WOMEN KNOW ABOUT MAMMOGRAPHY SCREENING?

While the debate about the benefits, or lack thereof, continues, the decision about if, or when, to have a mammogram ultimately should be made by each woman. But, in order for women to be active participants in the decision-making process and in order for women to make an informed decision about mammography screening, they need to better understand the range of uncertainties for both the potential benefits and the potential harms of mammography. Unfortunately, many women are not well informed about these issues. Common misconceptions about mammogram screening include (1) screening tests are meant for patients with known symptoms, (2) early detection is always a benefit, (3) screening reduces the incidence of breast cancer, and (4) all breast cancers progress.[20]

A telephone survey of random samples of women residing in the United States, the United Kingdom, Italy, and Switzerland, for example, found that a high proportion of women overestimated the benefits of screening mammography.[21] Most of the women polled seemed to be poorly informed about the likely benefit of screening, with misconceptions more prevalent among women in the United Kingdom and Italy. What this study's findings seem to imply is that women need better information about mammography screening.

Part of the problem is that women receive inaccurate or conflicting messages about the benefits of screening. Misleading "facts" about reduction in breast cancer mortality attributed to mammography are found in newspaper articles and on the Internet. Few articles discuss the implications of false positive and false negative results, and even fewer give information on adverse effects.[22] An honest and clear delineation of the range of outcomes of screening needs to be given to women before they are able to make an informed decision about mammography screening. One study looking at the information presented on the Internet by major interest groups (professional advocacy groups, consumer organizations, and governmental organizations) found that the Web sites hosted by professional advocacy groups and governmental organizations were "information poor" and severely biased in favor of screening.[23] The material provided by consumer organizations, however, was more comprehensive and balanced.

There is a need for objective information to be conveyed in a way that women can make informed decisions. Given current misconceptions about screening and given the quality of information available on the Internet and in the media, strategies at improving public understanding need to be formulated. A key question in the mammography debate, however, remains unanswered: How can public understanding be improved if the scientific community does not agree on the potential benefits of screening mammography? Unfortunately, there is no good answer to this question at this time. Many in the scientific community agree to disagree on the benefits of mammography screening. Among those who believe that mammography screening is beneficial, there are disagreements regarding what age screening should be started and how frequently it should be done.

The following is a brief summary of breast cancer screening recommendations and guidelines. These guidelines have changed over the years, and will probably continue to be updated as new evidence is made available.

## American Cancer Society

The ACS regards mammography screening as the gold standard. Other emerging technologies used alone are not appropriate for breast cancer screening but may be used in conjunction with mammography. The ACS recommends that *most women* begin annual mammography screening at age forty. What constitutes "most women"? The ACS suggests that women of average risk (no strong family history of breast cancer; do not carry one of the breast cancer genes) have annual mammography starting at age forty. For women age sixty-nine and over, the ACS suggests that the decision to continue with regular mammogram screening should be left to the woman in consultation with her physician. As long as she is in good health and could, if necessary, be a candidate for cancer treatment, mammography would be warranted. The ACS acknowledges that women with chronic health problems, serious illness, or a short life expectancy may not get the same benefit from screening as healthy women.

For those women who are high risk, consideration of starting screening earlier than age forty is suggested. More frequent mammograms may be warranted, and the addition of ultrasound, MRI, or digital mammography could be considered, even though the evidence currently available is not sufficient to justify these modalities as regular screening procedures.[24]

The ACS 2003 guidelines for breast cancer screening further advise women in their twenties and thirties to have CBEs as part of their routine physical examination (at least every three years). At age forty, clinical breast exams should be done annually. Regarding BSEs, the ACS does not feel that it is a realistic screening technique and that there is too much variability in the way breast tissue feels. But, if doing a BSE makes a woman more aware of the feel and texture of her breast, and if she thinks that she feels something different, then to that extent, the self-exam is useful.

## U.S. Preventive Services Task Force

The U.S. Preventive Services Task Force (USPSTF) is the leading independent panel of private-sector experts in prevention and primary care. It conducts rigorous and impartial assessments of scientific evidence for a broad range of preventive services. The USPSTF has stated that mammography is the best way to detect breast cancer in its earliest, most treatable stage. In 1989 and 1996, it endorsed mammography for women over age fifty, but in 2002, it extended that recommendation to all women over age forty, acknowledging that the strongest evidence of benefit and reduced mortality from breast cancer is among women aged fifty to sixty-nine. For women aged forty to forty-nine, evidence that screening mammography reduces mortality from breast cancer is weaker than that for women aged fifty to fifty-nine. The USPSTF stated that it is difficult to determine the incremental benefit of beginning screening at age forty rather than age fifty. Nevertheless, understanding that a woman's breast cancer risk increases over her lifetime, it advocates that women over forty consider having a mammogram every one to two years. For women seventy years and older, the recommendation is to have a mammogram every 1–2 years unless a woman has other serious illnesses that are likely to reduce her life expectancy.[25] The USPSTF acknowledges that the strongest evidence of benefit and reduced mortality from breast cancer is among women ages fifty to sixty-nine.

USPSTF understands that there are risks associated with mammography, notably false positive results that lead to further testing, but these risks lessen as a woman ages. Regarding routine CBEs and BSEs, the USPSTF notes that there is insufficient evidence to recommend for or against these methods as effective breast cancer screening methods.

Regarding screening intervals, the task force concluded that for women aged fifty or older, there was little evidence to suggest that annual mammography is more effective than mammography done every other year. For women aged forty to forty-nine, the available evidence does not show a clear advantage of annual mammography over biannual mammography. The age at which to recommend discontinuation of screening is not clear and the USPSTF did not make a recommendation.

## National Cancer Institute

After consideration of the scientific literature, the National Cancer Institute acknowledges the uncertainties and disagreements of the findings published. It recommends that women in their forties be screened every one to two years with mammography. Women aged fifty and older should be screened every one to two years as well, but those who are at higher than average risk of breast cancer should discuss with their physician when and how frequently mammography screening should be done.[26]

## Professional Organizations

All of the professional associations support mammography screening, although they vary in the recommended age at which to begin screening, the interval for screening, and the role of CBE. The differences in guidelines reflect a difference in the interpretation of the data. Some support screening with mammography beginning at age forty (American Medical Association, American College of Radiology, American College of Obstetricians and Gynecologists), while others recommend starting at age fifty (American Academy of Family Physicians, American College of Preventive Medicine) although women who are at high risk should begin screening at age forty.[27]

## IT IS A PERSONAL DECISION

The current debate makes the situation appear muddled. Some advocate mammography for all women, some have doubts about mammography screening's benefits for the younger and the older woman, and some say that mammography screening has no benefit for any woman regardless of age. The data are certainly showing mixed signals, but in epidemiology, nothing is clear-cut.

What is clear is that most women will *not* develop breast cancer in their lifetimes, although reading the statistics certainly gives a different impression of the odds. Breast cancer and breast cancer mortality continue to rise in the United States, and as the baby-boom generation enters their fifties and sixties, this trend most likely will persist. The technology to detect and diagnose breast cancer is more sophisticated and accurate now than in the past, but mammography, with its flaws, remains the most cost-effective, accurate means to screen for breast cancer on a large scale. Until there is a way to predict with greater confidence who is most at risk, mammography screening and CBEs are the best available strategies for detection of breast cancer at an early stage.

The odds that any individual woman will develop breast cancer do increase with age. The data are quite clear on this point. However, epidemiology deals with probabilities, and there is no way to predict or to know the precise age at which the benefits from screening mammography will be most effective. Each individual will have to make a subjective judgment as to when to begin screening and how frequently to schedule the screening. The precise age at which to discontinue screening mammography is also uncertain. Because risk for breast cancer increases with age, mammography screening could be important for many women. However, some older women (those in their seventies, for example) will probably die from other causes before screening detects a breast cancer. Until more effective screening techniques are developed, the most prudent course of action is for each woman, in consultation with her doctor, is to assess her potential risks and make a decision when to begin mammography screening. There are many private and personal factors that will influence a woman's decision when to have her first mammogram and whether she will have an annual screening or screening at less frequent intervals.

From a policy perspective, there are many unanswered questions. Do the imperfections of the trials invalidate or negate the importance of their findings? Trend data show that over the decades, breast cancer mortality has been declining. Is this decline a result of better detection and treatment? For those whose cancer was detected at an early, more treatable stage, the answer would most probably be a resounding *yes*. The costs (economic and emotional) associated with additional tests to work up suspicious lesions are not insignificant. There is no way to put a price on the anxiety and uncertainty a woman experiences as she waits for the pathology results. Women may render moot the debate over mammogram screening by electing to have mammograms, regardless of age, primarily to allay their own fears regardless of what the government or professional organizations or researchers recommend. Until there is more of a consensus among epidemiologists and clinicians, the debate will continue.

Women often have an unreal perception of their risk for breast cancer. For some, mammogram screening is a way to "be sure" that everything is okay. Peace of mind cannot and should not be discounted in the debate. For others, ignorance is bliss. The potential harms of screening appear to outweigh the potential benefits. For others, there is an educational or an economic issue discouraging her to be screened. Certainly an individual's perspective on the benefits and harms of screening, as well as her age, ethnicity, and values, will determine how often, if at all, she will have a mammogram. As such, there is a need for individualized guidance. If a woman believes that she is at increased risk, the way she and her physician approach screening will be different from that among women who are not at high risk for breast cancer. Physicians need to discuss the issue with their patients, and the patient needs to discuss her thoughts and her fears candidly. The importance of doctor–patient communication cannot be minimized, nor should it be ignored, in the debate over mammography screening.

## CHANGING ADVICE ON MAMMOGRAPHY

1963    HIP mammography trial begins.

1971    HIP study shows that mammography reduces breast cancer deaths by 30%.

1973    Wives of the president and vice president undergo mastectomies for breast cancer. Awareness of breast cancer and breast cancer screening is heightened.

1977–83    Four large-scale randomized controlled trials begin in Europe. Findings show that mammography decreases the breast cancer death rate by up to 30%.

Two Canadian trials find no benefit of mammography screening for women in their 40s, and find a clinical breast exam equally effective for women over age 50.

1979    A National Institutes of Health conference recommends annual mammography screening for women 50 and older. For women under age 50, it recommends screening only if they have had cancer or have a family history of it.

1980s    Sharp debate among organizations regarding screening recommendations. All recommend annual screening for women age 50 and older; some, including the National Institutes of Health, recommend screening for women in their 40s. Eleven national health-care organizations recommend an initial baseline mammogram for women age 35–39.

1992    The American Cancer Society drops its recommendation for baseline mammogram screening for women 35–39.

1993    National Cancer Institute drops its recommendation for screening women in their 40s.

1997    The National Institutes of Health conference concludes that there is not enough evidence to recommend routine screening for women in their 40s. The U.S. Senate gets involved in the debate and encourages a National Institutes of Health advisory board to reject the conference's recommendation. The Institute again recommends mammography screening for women in their 40s every 1 to 2 years.

The American Cancer Society recommends annual mammography screening for all women over age 40.

2000    A Danish study calls into question the methodology and findings of published trials and concludes that mammography screening's value may be overstated.

2001    After reassessing their data, the same Danish researchers again assert that screening mammography does not indicate any survival benefit for breast cancer, regardless of age. Political uproar ensues.

2002    Swedish researchers looking at the contribution of mammography screening to reductions in mortality conclude that screening can make a difference in survival. Other Swedish researchers find statistically significant reduction in breast cancer mortality.

The U.S. Preventive Services Task Force extended its recommendation for mammography screening every 1 to 2 years to women over age 40.

The National Cancer Institute recommends that women starting in their 40s have a mammogram every 1 to 2 years.

2003    The American Cancer Society regards screening mammography as the gold standard. It recommends that most women begin annual mammography screening at age 40. At age 69, the decision to continue with regular screening should be left to the woman in consultation with her physician. Women at high risk could start screening earlier than age 40. Women in their 20s and 30s should have regular clinical breast exams.

Source: Kolata, G and Moss M. X-Ray Vision in Hindsight: Science, Politics, and the Mammogram. New York Times. February 11, 2002.

## WEB SITES FOR FURTHER INFORMATION

http://www.cancer.gov/cancer_information/cancer_type/breast/
http://www.cancer.org
http://www.nbcam.org
http://www.fda.gov/cdrh/mammography/index.html
http://www.ahcpr.gov/clinic/3rduspstf/breastcancer

## CHAPTER 8

# Communicating with Doctors

## David Hyman and Madelon L. Finkel

W e have seen how technical and how technology-driven medicine is today. The main interaction between doctor and patient is about which test to order, what procedure to perform, and which drug to prescribe. Given all the high-tech advances, it is instructive to re-member that an important part of medicine is listening to the patient describe his or her symptoms, concerns, fears. Sure a test will confirm or rule out a diagnosis, but ordering that test was based on asking questions and listening. In short, despite the emergence of sophisticated technologies used to screen, diagnose, and treat disease, communication between doctor and patient is a primary tool for information exchange and decision making.

Are doctors good at listening to their patients? Probably not as good as they should be. Today's medical school curriculum includes courses on teaching medical students how to listen. The students are taught to pay attention to what their patients are saying and to understand how their own emotions affect perceptions and maybe even their clinical practice. It probably is impossible to teach or train someone to be empathetic. But, it is possible to help an individual relate better to another by listening.

Doctors need to understand that patients seek guidance from them, and, as such, doctors need to embrace and encourage the patient to be an active participant in her own care. Unfortunately, it is frequently heard that patients feel that their doctor is not listening to them, is ignoring their concerns, or is not taking what they are saying seriously. For many patients, there can be a distressing lack of communication.

Studies have linked physicians' communication skills to a variety of positive and negative outcomes.[1] Positive outcomes include high patient satisfaction, higher levels of adherence to treatment regimens, and better physical and mental health status. Poor communication affects a host of factors such as patient participation in treatment decision making, patient compliance with treatment, and patient satisfaction with medical care. Poor doctor–patient communication can lead to unnecessary misunderstandings that promote distrust, anger, and possibly even legal action. Most important, constructive doctor–patient relationships are associated with better health outcomes such as improved blood-sugar control in diabetics, blood pressure reduction in hypertensive patients, and, having annual or biannual mammograms.

Physician gender is an important component in the doctor–patient relationship. Differences in the interpersonal style of women compared to men are well documented. The female physician, for example, might facilitate a more open exchange than a male physician. One large-scale review found that female physicians engage in significantly more active partnership behaviors, positive talk, psychological counseling, and emotionally focused talk than male physicians.[2] There was no difference in the amount or quality of clinical information given, however. The female physician also tends to have longer visits than their male counterparts. While nobody is advocating that female physicians make better doctors than male physicians, or that one should only seek care from a female physician, the point is that there are differences in doctor–patient communication depending on the gender of the physician. Of course there are plenty of insensitive female physicians, just as there are plenty of male physicians who are excellent communicators.

Of course, it is in the best interests of both doctors and patients that each party understands the importance of listening and communicating. For doctors, this understanding will help equip them to meet the therapeutic and emotional needs of their patients. For patients, this understanding will encourage them to share important information and to articulate questions and concerns with their doctors. The emotional gravity of cancer contributes unique stresses as well as added importance to the doctor–patient relationship.

## ONCOLOGY AND THE DOCTOR–PATIENT RELATIONSHIP

The shifting paradigm from inpatient to outpatient cancer care has put today's cancer patients in a position of increased responsibility for monitoring and managing their disease and its treatment.[3] Because most cancer treatment now is done in an ambulatory setting, doctors must rely increasingly on the cancer patient's self-reporting to manage and to adjust treatment regimens. Patients, on the other hand, must rely increasingly on themselves or family members/friends, and not the hospital staff, to manage the sequelae of their disease and its treatment.

Despite the increasing importance of open communication in cancer care, the literature shows that cancer patients, in particular, have problems speaking with their doctors. One study found that a staggering 84 percent of breast cancer patients expressed some difficulties communicating with their medical team.[4] When asked more specifically about this, patients identify each of the following categories as particularly problematic: understanding their doctors, expressing feelings, maintaining a sense of control, and asking questions.

Cancer patients require significantly more information about their illness than do patients afflicted with other diseases. Women newly diagnosed with breast cancer have many questions. How far has the cancer has spread? What are my odds for a cure? What are my treatment options? How am I going to feel once I start treatment? Information can help cancer patients develop a sense of mastery over their illness. This sense of power extends not only to their disease but also to their relationships with physicians. An overwhelming majority of cancer patients in the United States say that they do not want the information they receive about their disease to be censored.[5]

Given the huge variability in cancer patients (different age, ethnicity, socioeconomic background, and the like), issues and concerns will naturally vary. Younger women, for example, might be more concerned with issues of sexuality and physical attractiveness during and after treatment; older women might be more concerned about issues of self-care. Feelings of resignation, or "there is nothing I can do about my cancer," attitudes are more prevalent in certain ethnic groups, while others may approach cancer treatment as a battle to be won at all costs. The following quote from one breast cancer patient sums up what many patients feel:

> There's a feeling that they [professionals] have an enormous amount of information and the patient has very little. That creates a kind of a power thing. It can become more of a partnership . . . because the patient needs more information rather than less. But I think they [professionals] tend to be very conservative with the information and say "let's only give patients so much." They [professionals] don't want to confuse patients. . . . I want it to be more like the other side. That is give patients quite a bit of information; we need more rather than less.[6]

The diagnosis of cancer can be devastating. More than any other illness, cancer evokes fears of pain, disfigurement, and despair. Even the suspicion of cancer can provoke anxiety and fear. Women investigated for abnormal breast findings later found to be benign (false positives) often experience sustained emotional distress from the scare. Women diagnosed with breast cancer may experience a sense of alienation, decreased self-esteem, hopelessness, anxiety, depression, hostility, and guilt. These feelings can last for years after treatment.[7] Diminished sexual function and poor body image are two of the most common and difficult to treat consequences of breast cancer therapy.

Even among women who undergo lumpectomy, the psychosocial impact and sexual sequelae can be significant. In patients who survive their initial bout with breast cancer, the fear of recurrence can become a life-long burden and can accentuate the distress caused by even the most minor physical ailment. The diagnosis of breast cancer can also cause significant anxiety for the patient's immediate support network. Family members often experience mood swings and feel depressed, angry, and helpless. Husbands often report many of the same emotional issues as their wives. If there are young children, the emotional tension can be extremely high, for obvious reasons.

Research has begun to look more closely at whether good doctor–patient communication can improve mental and psychical health outcomes. It is now fairly well accepted that strong doctor–patient relationships can help improve a patient's mental health outcomes.[8] Doctors who show interest in and acceptance and understanding of their patients generally have patients who have less anxiety and other psychological difficulties coping with their cancer. Is sum, it stands to reason that effective communication between doctor and patient is the key to good care, cancer or otherwise.

## NAVIGATING THE MEDICAL TEAM

The medical team of the twenty-first century in charge of caring for breast cancer patients often includes an internist, medical oncologist, radiation oncologist, breast surgeon, social worker, physician's assistant, nurse, medical technician, and office administrator. Navigating this daunting array of health-care professionals can be both confusing and stressful for the patient. As a result, breast cancer patients often perceive a lack of continuity in their care that can undermine relationship building and interfere with information exchange. One patient relates her experience:

> I began to feel like a number or nameless person or a cancer patient. I felt like there wasn't any recognition of individuality. There was a protocol that was followed, and everyone was more or less given the same treatment, and I just kind of subjected myself to it. I didn't feel that I received very much from it...I felt a bit patronized or condescended to.[9]

Successfully navigating the medical team requires that patients understand the different roles of doctors and nurses. Patients most often interact with their doctor during the physical examination. The physician takes a history by asking the patient a number of (usually yes or no) questions regarding her health and that of immediate family members, inquires about any troubling symptoms, performs a physical, and, if available, reviews laboratory results. Patients asked about this type of encounter relate that they often feel hesitant to ask questions of their physicians; many patients are intimidated by the "doctor knows best" mentality. Patients most often interact with the nurse before and after the exam or when blood is drawn. The nurse is generally viewed as a sympathetic figure who listens and focuses on the patient's emotional needs. During cancer treatment, it is the nurse who supports and comforts the patient during therapy. Often patients identify nurses as key advocates and interpreters on the medical team. Patients see their nurses as particularly adept at facilitating productive interactions between themselves and their doctor. Summarizes one patient:

> I feel confident that if I phone up and just get the nurse, well she very often has the answer. She seems interested in knowing how I am coping. She listens to everything I have to say and answers my questions. If she doesn't have the answer then she goes and asks the doctor and calls me back.[10]

## THINGS THAT CAN GO WRONG

A number of factors can contribute to strained doctor–patient communication during breast cancer treatment. Physicians who care for cancer patients may themselves experience tremendous psychological distress. Oncologists are constantly managing relationships with patients who are experiencing devastating, serious, and potentially fatal diseases. As a result, oncologists may try to achieve emotional self-preservation by maintaining a professional detachment from their patients. Distancing tactics can damage the relationship of the physician with both the patient and the patient's family. Doctors' personal feelings of unease or anxiety over the uncertainties of cancer care also may influence the amount of information given to their patients. For example, a physician may mistake her own anxiety over death and end-of-life care as being the patient's viewpoint, and may thus avoid broaching the subject with a terminally ill patient. The doctor's feelings of powerlessness or failure may create an awkward, distant relationship to develop. On the other hand, crisis situations may bring out the best in the medical team and strengthen the bond between the patient and the doctor. The key is for all players to talk to each other and to let each one be as honest as possible about the treatment and the prognosis.

The different languages spoken by doctors and their patients may also create a number of communication barriers. Physicians are bilingual; they speak both everyday language and medical language. Though doctors often feel that they are speaking in everyday language to their patients, patients may not always perceive this. In an attempt to compensate, many cancer patients try to learn and use medical language. Patients, however, can only partially master the thousands of confusing medical terms, and potentially significant misinterpretations can arise.

In addition to explaining the medical aspects of disease to the patient, the physician will need to explain the risks of treatment. Effective risk communication is the basis for informed patient consent for medical treatment; yet, few physicians receive formal training in communicating risk. There are many different dimensions and inherent uncertainties that need to be taken into account.[11] The physician needs to understand that most patients may not be able to digest most of the information, and emotions rather than facts probably will cloud the issue. The physician should help the patient understand risks by displaying both a competent and caring approach.[12] Clearly, the way a physician communicates risk can affect a patient's perception of risks.

In addition to the gender and age of the patient and the physician, cultural differences can create significant barriers to communication between doctors and their patients.[13] Cultural background often shapes a patient's perspective on disease, especially cancer. Sociocultural mores often shape the way patients perceive their physicians and how they interact with the health-care team. The cultural background of both the doctor and the patient can and does influence the way that each views and interacts with the other. Cultural sensitivity is therefore an essential prerequisite for the establishment effective doctor–patient relationships.

## IS THERE A BETTER WAY?

The difficulty in maintaining the continuity of doctor–patient relations in the context of the multidisciplinary medical team has led many clinicians and researchers to look for better ways to provide care for breast cancer patients. In part, their work has focused on developing "one-stop" clinics designed to shorten the amount of time and number of visits it takes for a women to be diagnosed with breast cancer. These clinics can investigate abnormal breast findings by offering patients a CBE, ultrasound scan, cytology, and mammography in one visit. The tests are read while the patient waits, and results are given on the same day. The proliferation of one-stop breast cancer centers attests to the profession's awareness of the tremendous emotional stress that can accompany the prediagnostic phase of breast cancer treatment. Though studies of these one-stop centers have found that they often help patient anxiety and streamline patient care, the cost effectiveness of these centers remains in question.[14]

Medical centers around the world have also invested heavily in collaborative interdisciplinary breast cancer specialty centers that operate out of one location to provide an integrated treatment experience for the patient. These centers offer patients the ability to be cared for by a team of physicians accustomed to working together. This model facilitates improved medical team interactions.

## THE IMPORTANCE OF PATIENT SATISFACTION

Concomitant with an open and comfortable communication relationship, patient satisfaction is another important component in the doctor–patient relationship. It may seem intuitive to anyone who has been to the doctor that satisfaction with one's doctor can strongly influence the quality of the health-care experience. It is well understood that patient satisfaction is strongly influenced by the esteem in which patients hold their doctors. Since it is sometimes difficult for a nonclinician to assess the clinical expertise of a physician, patients sometimes judge the competence of their doctors based on the quality of the physician's interpersonal skills. In particular, physicians who take the time to listen, to answer questions, to show that "they care," are viewed as being a "good doctor."

Physicians' affective behaviors are also strongly predictive of patient satisfaction.[15] Affective behaviors include tone of voice and other nonverbal cues such as posture. Together they communicate physician attitude and state of mind (i.e., nervousness, irritation, friendliness, and attentiveness). Cancer patients are hungry for information. They also are thus exquisitely sensitive to nonverbal communication because they perceive it as a form of additional information. As a result, verbal/nonverbal mismatch on the part of physicians can be perceived as a lack of genuineness and can lead to patient dissatisfaction.

## THE IMPORTANCE OF PATIENT COMPLIANCE

Research has also studied the affects of strong doctor–patient relationships on patient compliance. In general, the likelihood that a patient will comply with instructions is a function of the patient's perceived benefits of the intervention weighed against the costs and potential side effects of the treatment. Patient compliance with cancer treatment is not the same as that for a chronic or acute disease. In cancer care, most treatments (surgery, chemotherapy, or radiation) are performed in the doctor's office or hospital. Also, cancer is a symptomatic disease, and not complying with treatment can lead quickly to severe morbidity and death. Partially because of this, good doctor–patient relationships have not been strongly correlated with better compliance in the cancer setting. Poor doctor–patient communication and a lack of trust in the doctor's judgment, however, can lead cancer patients to seek alternative, nontraditional, cancer therapies. While some physicians may view this as a form of noncompliance, had there been a more open line of communication, perhaps the patient would have felt more comfortable discussing alternative treatments. By not telling the doctor about reliance on nontraditional therapies, potentially serious adverse events can occur.

## IS THE PATIENT LISTENING?

Patient recall and comprehension of instructions given by physicians in the medical encounter is know to be generally poor. In the primary-care setting, patients interviewed about the content of their visit demonstrate confusion about what their physician told them between 7 and 47 percent of the time, depending on the complexity of the information covered. In the cancer setting, studies have shown that patients register little to no information immediately after being told they have cancer. It is therefore important that physicians tailor the information they provide during the initial consultation. A physician who goes into a lengthy discourse of treatment options and prognosis with a newly diagnosed cancer patient is wasting his time. Indeed, such an interaction is usually going to be counterproductive because the information the patient can digest at that time is limited. All the patient hears and remembers is that she has cancer. As such, patients may benefit tremendously by having a family member or close friend with them. This individual can provide emotional support as well as listen and take notes on what the doctor is saying.

Verification techniques are an invaluable, often overlooked tool for improving patient comprehension.[16] Physicians can verify that their patients have correctly understood them by asking them to restate the information in their own words. Similarly, patients can verify information they have received by reiterating it and asking their physicians to correct any misunderstandings. Verification avoids many of the miscommunications that can result when a patient tries to translate "doctor speak" to everyday language. Patient recall and comprehension can be significantly improved by a strong doctor–patient relationship and by using verification techniques.

## POWER-SHARING AND DECISION MAKING IN THE DOCTOR–PATIENT RELATIONSHIP

The approach to power-sharing and decision making in the doctor–patient relationship is something relatively new in medicine. Historically, doctors saw themselves as father figures (most of the physicians were males not so long ago) whose responsibility it was to act as the patient's guardian, articulating and implementing what they believed was best for the patient. The "paternalistic" physician presented information in a selective manner that encouraged the patient to assent to the doctor's desired intervention. This model assumed that the patient would eventually be grateful for the decisions made by the physician, even if the patient was unlikely to have consented to or even understood them at the time.

In 1984, Jay Katz wrote *The Silent World of the Doctor and Patient*, in which he argued compassionately for the ability of patients to participate in treatment decisions.[17] In his book, Dr. Katz relates the story of Iphigenia Jones, a breast cancer patient he met while attending a panel discussion. Jones was an attractive, twenty-one-year-old single woman who had developed a malignant breast lesion. Her surgeon strongly believed that breast-conserving surgery with radiation was an inferior treatment and scheduled her for a mastectomy without discussing the alternatives, as was common practice at the time. In the days leading up to the surgery, however, Jones's surgeon became increasingly anxious about performing a grossly scarring procedure with such a young, attractive woman. The night before the surgery, striking out new ethical territory, he had a conversation with Jones in which he defended his belief in mastectomy as the superior treatment but discussed with her other breast-conserving options. Jones immediately postponed the mastectomy and, after taking time to educate herself, eventually opted for lumpectomy with radiation.

Today, doctors are expected to be much more forthcoming with patients concerning both their condition and treatment options. The shift from paternalism in the medical encounter to a system that encourages active patient participation has been widely hailed as an important improvement in the way doctors and patients communicate. This development is consistent with the value changes in our society that now uphold the importance of self-sovereignty in medical decision making. While several studies have supported the value of this thinking, until recently, much less has been known about how this model functions in the context of the cancer clinic. Do cancer patients share the same desire to participate in medical decision making?

The two main models for modern medical decision making are the *doctor-centered approach* and the *patient-centered approach*. The doctor-centered approach affirms that the doctor is an expert adviser whose task it is to incorporate the values of her patient when making treatment recommendations.[18] The physician elicits the patient's values as part of the medical encounter. However, the point is the patient's values can be difficult to determine, open to interpretation, and easily influenced by the physician's own set of values.

The patient-centered approach affirms the doctor as a vehicle for enabling the patient to express all of her reasons for coming. These reasons include all dimensions of the patient's illness, including symptoms, thoughts, feelings, impact on function, and expectations of the visit. The egalitarian nature of this approach means that the patient must play an active role in the decision-making process. The doctor allows for a mutual discussion of the relevant problems as the patient has identified them and provides an opportunity for the patient to ask clarifying questions concerning the proposed treatment and management plan. The doctor also takes into account the patient's family, and social and religious factors. This is especially important in the care of breast cancer. A thirty-five-year-old mother with young children is very likely to have different concerns and expectations about her breast cancer therapy than an older woman who has already raised her family. While each has concerns and fears, their perspective is probably different because of their different stage in life.

One study aimed at determining decision-making preferences interviewed 1,000 women with breast cancer and asked them whether they wanted an active, collaborative, or passive role in choosing their treatment. Twenty-two percent wanted active roles, 44 percent wanted collaborative roles, and 34 percent wanted passive roles. Overall, however, only 42 percent of the women achieved their desired level of participation.[19] In other words, doctors appear to be poor judges of their patients' preferences for control. Moreover, women who desired passive roles were the most likely to achieve their desired level of control, indicating that doctors are still more willing to assume control than relinquish it.

In this study, the best predictor of control preference was education; those with higher levels of education wanted more control. In addition, women in the oldest age bracket (over seventy) were one-fifth as likely to want active roles as women in the youngest age bracket (under fifty). Other studies have indicated that sociodemographic variables such as education, age, marital status, and ethnicity are weak predictors of decision-making preference. The controversial influence of these factors in determining patients' preferences for decision making means that doctors should be wary of stereotyping their patients based on these characteristics.

Given the heterogeneous decision-making preferences of women, it is clear that no single power dynamic will suit all patients. One study found that while two-thirds of patients prefer a patient-centered approach to care, a significant minority of one-third prefers a doctor-centered approach.[20] There is no one-size-fits-all solution; doctors must tailor each relationship based on patient preference. In so doing, patients must verbalize her preferences. There must be a dialogue in order for the relationship to be mutually beneficial.

Studies that have looked at women at different stages of therapy and disease have shown that health status strongly influences the decision-making preferences for women with breast cancer. One such study surveyed women without breast disease, women with benign breast growths, and women with malignant growths for their various decision-making preferences.[21] The healthy women wanted most control, whereas the women with benign masses and women with malignant masses wanted increasingly less control. In a related finding, one major study raised the concern that some women in the end-stages of breast cancer are being pressed to assume more active decision-making roles than they desire.[22] Hence, for some, the more life-threatening the cancer, the more passive a decision-making role the patient desires.

For the most part, cancer patients have a strong desire for information. How active a partner in decision making the woman elects to be is another story. The desire for more information is sometimes confused with a presumed wish to participate in clinical decision making. The important message is that doctors must not assume that because a patient asks a lot of questions, she wishes to play an equally active role in decision making.

## SHARED DECISION MAKING

What then, is the ideal model for decision making in the doctor–patient relationship? Research suggests that a combination of the doctor-centered and patient-centered models may be the most productive approach to decision making in breast cancer care. In this model, the patient leads in areas where she is an expert (her symptoms, preferences, and concerns) and the doctor leads in areas where he/she is an expert (the details of disease and treatment options). Studies measuring patient satisfaction demonstrate the best outcomes when patients participate in shared decision-making relationships with their physicians.[23] Moreover, the same study found that increasing trust in one's doctor is associated with an increased desire to participate in decision making. A strong doctor–patient relationship can encourage patients to share in their own decision making, an arrangement that is associated with the highest level of patient satisfaction.

How can physicians encourage patients to participate in shared decision making while simultaneously respecting their patients' expressed preferences for control? A simple solution is for doctors to listen and to encourage their patients to ask questions. Unfortunately, many physicians do a poor job of eliciting their patients' questions and concerns. One study that used audiotaped internal medicine consultations found that physicians either interrupted or failed to elicit their patients' chief concern in three out of four encounters.[24] The same study showed that physicians interrupted their patients an average of eighteen seconds after the beginning of the medical encounter.

Doctors may feel that the era of managed care does not permit spending much time talking to a patient. Some may feel that allowing patients to express their concerns fully would "take too long." Interestingly, it has been documented that patients who were allowed to finish speaking never took more than 150 seconds. By encouraging patients to ask questions and allowing them sufficient time to finish their thought, doctors in effect allow their patients to control the duration of the consultation, the topics covered, and the level of detail discussed. Question asking is a relationship building exercise that encourages trust and promotes shared medical decision making.

## TECHNIQUES FOR IMPROVING COMMUNICATION— WHAT CAN PATIENTS DO?

Certain patient behaviors contribute positively to doctor–patient communication. In particular, patients who demonstrate a measured degree of assertiveness in the medical encounter often build stronger, more productive relationships with their physicians. The physician sees assertiveness as a sign that the patient wishes to be an active participant in her care. Patients who are assertive benefit from a sense of control and self-determination often not shared by their less-assertive peers. One patient offers the following perspective:

> I'd say I'm assertive but not necessarily aggressive.... I give people a lot of leeway but I don't take no for an answer, and I don't take a brush-off for an answer. I think it's something I've worked on because you know, we're talking about my life.[25]

Patients who engage in active question asking are also more likely to build strong relationships with their physicians. Patients who ask more questions get more answers, and these answers help patients better adjust to living with their disease. Similarly, patients who research breast cancer outside of the office (and have physicians who are willing to acknowledge and encourage this behavior) can build strong relationships with their doctor. In the current health-care environment, the time spent with the doctor is often insufficient to discuss treatment options and patient concerns. Patients who conduct their own research become better informed about their disease and, as a result, are better able to communicate with their physicians. Comments one patient:

> My experience has been that, if you want to have better communication, you have to be better informed ... you can't go in expecting the doctors or the nurses to solve all the problems and have all the answers. I think you make it easier for the professional if you take it on yourself to learn something about your chemotherapy.[26]

Over the past ten years an increasing amount of attention has been devoted to developing skills workshops designed specifically to improve on the ability of cancer patients to communicate their unique needs and concerns to their physicians. Many of these techniques can be learned or practiced in informal settings with untrained facilitators, such as family or friends. One meta-analysis of over sixty-two different psychosocial interventions in adult cancer patients found that they improved patients' emotional adjustment, functional adjustment, treatment- and disease-related symptoms, and global outcomes. Overall, each category improved by roughly 20 percent, a statistically and clinically significant amount. Not every method will be appropriate for every patient or accepted by every doctor. A number of these interventions are presented here as examples.

Providing patients with audiotapes of consultations has been one of the most widely studied methods for improving doctor–patient communication in the cancer clinic. In particular, one systematic review analyzed the results of eight controlled studies that looked at the outcomes of providing patients with audiotapes of their consultations, accompanied with or without written summaries. Between 83 and 96 percent of the patients in these studies found the recordings and/or summaries helpful. Seventy-five percent of these patients indicated that the audiotape improved their understanding and recall of the consultation without creating further new anxiety.[27]

Of the four studies that looked at the affect of the tapes on satisfaction, two found significant improvement. Although none of the studies demonstrated statistically significant effects on patient anxiety, 83 percent of the patients that took home an audiotape listened to it. Moreover, 68 percent of these patients played the tape for others, usually a spouse. In fact, patients' families may be the group that most benefits from taped records of their loved ones' consultations.[28]

Family members often have tremendous difficulty trying to monitor the progress of their relative during treatment. As mentioned previously, patients have poor recall of their consultations and often find it difficult to recount their doctor visits with family members. Patients may also be reluctant to relive their visits because it causes anxiety. Audiotapes help family members feel as if they are in the doctor's office with their loved ones during the consultation. Patients who speak English as a second language or elderly patients who may not understand or remember what the doctor said also can benefit from audiotapes. These recordings enable the patient with or without family support to study what the doctor said during the consultation.[29]

Although it may not be common practice for oncologists to audiotape consultations, patients should feel comfortable asking their physicians' permission to tape meetings themselves. Oncologists are becoming increasingly accepting of having a tape recorder with them in the examination room. However, if the doctor is uncomfortable, a related approach is to bring a family member or close friend along to the consultation. The companion can act as both an emotional support and note-taker.

The utility of consultation planning sessions has also been studied. In general, the goals of these sessions are twofold. Consultation planning is designed to help the patient identify her main concerns regarding breast cancer and then facilitate her ability to express these concerns with her physician during the consultation. Often the final result of these sessions is the creation of a prompt sheet. Although the format may vary from a simple list to a well-developed flow chart, prompt sheets help ensure that the patient covers all of the concerns and questions that she determines to be important during the consultation planning session. Prompt sheets significantly reduce patient anxiety and consultation duration and improve patient recall when the physician acknowledges and accepts their presence. Despite the proven utility of prompt sheets, some physicians may feel threatened when their patients use them. This reaction is unproductive and can lead to strained or even adversarial interactions during the consultation. Hopefully, these physicians represent a small minority of current medical practitioners.

Prompt sheets can be developed in a number of different ways. In one research study, patient responses to a standardized questionnaire were

## Table 8.1
### Example of the Standardized Survey

1. How my upcoming consultation with Dr. A came about:
   I need to get rid of this lump.
   The biopsy did not yield clean margins, so I'm scheduled
      for more surgery.
2. What I will say and do during the consultation:
   I am ready to do what is necessary to save my life. Do I need to
      have a mastectomy?
   Am I a candidate for a lumpectomy?
   I want to go back to work as soon as possible.
   How can I minimize recovery time?
3. What I will be thinking or feeling but not sharing with the
      physician:
   I don't want to deal with the disfigurement of surgery.

Note: The survey helped patients reflect on their questions and concerns, especially ones that they might not feel comfortable raising with their physicians.

**Figure 8.1**
**Example of Flow Chart**

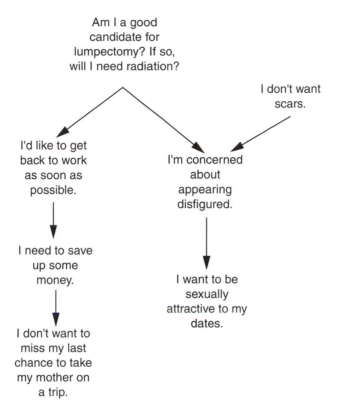

Am I a good candidate for lumpectomy? If so, will I need radiation?

I don't want scars.

I'd like to get back to work as soon as possible.

I'm concerned about appearing disfigured.

I need to save up some money.

I want to be sexually attractive to my dates.

I don't want to miss my last chance to take my mother on a trip.

used to construct a flow chart that could then be used as a prompt sheet (table 8.1 and figure 8.1).

A less-structured method of developing prompt sheets involves a facilitator who simply asks a patient to relate her past experiences and apprehensions regarding breast cancer and her interactions with physicians. The facilitator takes notes that can be used as a prompt sheet. Although this method requires little to no formal training, it is helpful in improving patients' ability to express their concerns during the medical encounter.[30]

Prompt sheets can also be a useful tool for doctors who are trying to improve communication with their patients. Some physicians ask their patients to write down and fax or e-mail a list of questions the patient has before each consultation. The questions are then included in the patient's chart and can be referred to by the doctor throughout the consultation to ensure that all concerns have been addressed.

The ability for patients to organize and express their thoughts and concerns in the medical encounter can be expanded on in sessions with trained psychologists or psychiatrists. Psychiatric referrals during cancer care, especially in those patients who are having significant difficulty coping with their illness, can have tremendous benefits. Patients should be encouraged to ask their physicians whether they could benefit from seeing a mental health-care professional during their treatment.

## SUMMARY

Maintaining an open dialogue between doctor and patient is particularly important in cancer care where the emotional strain on the patient can be severe. Despite this, the majority of breast cancer patients express difficulty in communicating with their physicians. In part, this difficulty might represent the failure of oncologists to meet the informational needs of their patients, which include detailed facts on diagnosis, prognosis, treatment options, and family risk. Good doctor–patient relationships can reduce the psychiatric morbidity experienced by breast cancer patients, which includes denial, anxiety, depression, and difficulty adjusting to living with cancer.

Patient satisfaction is strongly related to the quality of the doctor–patient relationship. More satisfied patients are less anxious over their treatment and adjust better to living with cancer. Many health-care professionals are involved in coordinating care, and, as a result, many patients perceive a lack of continuity in their care. In an effort to acknowledge this perception, integrated one-stop breast care centers are viewed as a means of facilitating coordinated care.

Patient recall and comprehension of what the doctor said can be a significant problem in cancer care. A number of interventions including bringing a note-taker, verification techniques, and tape-recording consultations can improve recall and comprehension.

Breast cancer patients have a diverse range of preferences regarding how active a role they wish to play when discussing and choosing treatment options. Whereas many desire to have a collaborative role in decision making, others are more comfortable in a more passive role. The ideal decision-making relationship could combine elements of the active, collaborative, and the passive models: the patient leads in areas where she is an expert (her symptoms, preferences, and concerns), and the doctor leads in areas where he/she is an expert (the details of the disease and treatment options). Doctors can promote this relationship by encouraging their patients to ask questions. In cases where the patient is having significant difficulty coping with her illness, mental health counseling is often helpful.

Certain patient behaviors as well as patient-centered interventions can be used to improve the therapeutic relationship. Being assertive, asking questions, and doing outside research were all identified by both patients and physicians as behaviors that can improve communication. Providing patients with audiotapes of consultation is an excellent means of improving patient recall, comprehension, and satisfaction of the medical encounter. In addition, family members and patients who speak English as a second language find the audiotapes particularly useful.

Consultation prepping with or without the accompanying use of prompt sheets can help facilitate doctor–patient communication. A patient can bring outlines generated by consultation prepping to the consultation to ensure that important points previously identified are addressed.

Both doctors and patients need to acknowledge the importance of communication in the doctor–patient relationship. Doctors must understand that, for the most part, today's patients want to be involved in some way in their treatment and care, and many patients come to the doctor's office well informed about their illness and the various treatment options. In turn, patients need to communicate to their doctor how active or passive a role they wish to take. Neither the doctor nor the patient is a mind reader.

## CHAPTER 9

# Coping with Breast Cancer

The diagnosis of an illness like cancer, with the fears attached to it and the threat of life itself, results in a complex set of issues that the individual must confront: physical symptoms (especially pain); psychological reactions of fear and sadness; concern for the family and their endangered future; facing the existential issues of life and death; and seeking a comforting philosophical, spiritual or religious belief system to help give a tolerable meaning to the new world of illness.[1]

Although there have been tremendous advances in cancer research that have led to increased survival (breast cancer is not an automatic death sentence), the emotional upheavals a diagnosis of breast cancer confers are not insignificant. For many women, it is a time of realization that one's life will never be the same. There is an acute awareness of one's vulnerability and mortality. Being told that one has breast cancer unleashes a cascade of emotions: disbelief, fear of death, anger, grief, vulnerability, denial, anxiety, and, in some, depression. A diagnosis of breast cancer connotes an uncertain future of medical procedures and tests. The impersonal and disfiguring treatments of surgery, chemotherapy, and radiation each have psychological ramifications. While surgery will leave a scar that in time will fade, the psychological sequela effects of being a breast cancer survivor may never disappear.

Most women with breast cancer report a host of psychological emotions. Fear of death, loss of a sense of control, changes in quality of life and interpersonal relationships are often cited by breast cancer patients. Suffice it to say that psychological distress among cancer patients is not insignificant. Unfortunately, only a small proportion of cancer patients who are clinically depressed or anxious are identified by their oncologist[2] and even fewer are referred for counseling or support.[3]

The psychological dimensions of adapting to a breast cancer diagnosis will naturally vary among individuals depending on many factors including type and stage of the disease and the type and length of time of treatment. Dealing with the initial shock of the diagnosis and the implications of the disease also will vary depending on coping skills, level of emotional maturity, personality characteristics, and social support networks. Breast cancer, which usually necessitates the removal of all or some of the breast, holds different psychological challenges compared to colon cancer, for example, the evidence of which is primarily internal, out of sight. Indeed, treating the cancer is comparatively easy compared to dealing with the psychological ramifications of the disease. At each stage of the disease, there are three basic psychosocial issues that a cancer patient faces:

1. The *diagnostic and treatment* stage demands recognition of the diagnosis of cancer. Denial, anger, fear, anxiety compete with each other and can affect the most emotionally strong. Coping with the realization that one has cancer, trying to make appropriate decisions, and enduring the insults of treatment is often stressful.
2. Treatment was successful, and the patient is in *remission* and now must attempt to resume a "normal" life. Returning to a normal life in terms of the individual's sense of self as well as interactions with family, friends, and wider social circles carries a degree of stress. It is not uncommon for a woman to experience feelings of increased anxiety when active treatment is completed. Periodic check-ups are constant reminders that there may be a risk of recurrence.
3. *Cancer recurrence* is the cruelest twist of fate. At this stage, there is most often a progression into the final stage of death and dying. Coping with this news, this setback, can test the most stalwart.

## IS THERE A "CANCER PERSONALITY"?

Are some individuals prone to get cancer because of who they are? Much has been written about Type A personality and heart disease. Is there such a thing for cancer patients? Is stress a risk factor for cancer? Are anxiety and depression risk factors? Not so long ago, it was thought that hostile arguing, for example, may compromise the immune function and thus make one more prone to cancer. Implicit in this is the belief that if one changed one's personality or behavior, one could avoid cancer.

A survey of almost four hundred breast cancer survivors sought to determine to what they attributed the cause of their breast cancer. Despite a lack of evidence substantiating stress as a cause of breast cancer, 42 percent of the respondents felt that stress was the cause of their cancer; one-quarter said that genetics or the environment or hormones was the cause (27 percent, 26 percent, and 24 percent, respectively). When asked what they thought prevented breast cancer recurrence (multiple responses were permitted), 60 percent felt that a positive attitude was responsible, 50 percent said diet, 40 percent indicated a healthy lifestyle/exercise, 28 percent cited stress reduction, 26 percent felt prayer prevented recurrence, and only 3.9 percent said that tamoxifen was responsible for preventing recurrence.[4]

Other studies that looked at psychosocial factors and their relationship with breast cancer have most often examined the role of personality and stress as risk factors in cancer. The role of psychosocial influences in the development of breast cancer has not been shown conclusively, but it should be noted that most of the studies are methodologically flawed, making specific pronouncements about any association difficult. One large-scale meta-analysis examining the relationship between psychosocial factors and the development of breast cancer, however, found only a modest association between specific psychosocial factors and breast cancer. There is little support that personality and stress influence the development of breast cancer, nor is there support that anxiety/depression or expression of anger contribute to the development of cancer.[5] The data seem to support the primacy of biology and genetics over personality in the development of breast cancer.

## COPING STYLES

It has been hypothesized that how a woman responds to and copes with her breast cancer has some influence on survival. That is, those individuals who exhibit a "will to live" and "fighting spirit" are thought to have an increased chance of survival. Some cancer patients who survive their disease often believe that there is a direct relationship between their psychological state and their long-term survival. Those who seem helpless or hopeless, who are having difficulty coping with their disease, are thought to have a poorer chance of survival. Some studies found that the presence of psychiatric symptoms was significantly related to poorer prognosis,[6] while other studies found no relation between psychiatric symptoms and disease outcome.[7]

One large study looking at the influence of psychological response on survival in breast cancer found that a high helplessness/hopelessness score had a moderate but detrimental effect on five-year event-free survival. A high score for depression was linked to a significantly reduced chance of survival. These individuals were more likely to have relapsed or died during the five years. But, neither was having a fighting spirit associated with improved survival.[8] Furthermore, a systematic review of published and unpublished prospective studies that focused on psychological coping styles of cancer patients and how these coping styles influenced or affected survival and recurrence found no significant associations with survival or recurrence by coping style. Neither fighting spirit nor hopelessness/helplessness were shown to play an important part in survival from or recurrence of cancer.[9]

Although research findings are mixed, no study looking at psychological factors and cancer survival was sufficiently rigorous to reach a definite conclusion. Many studies fail to control for important medical and demographic risk factors, which could inflate the importance of psychological factors in cancer survival. Small sample sizes compromise the ability to detect the affects of psychological factors. In some studies, the participants were self-selected, introducing bias to the findings. Also, the psychological measures used in the study are, to some degree, intercorrelated. Depression may be a psychological concomitant of subjective stress. Depressive symptoms and sense of control may also have a link. Clearly, factors other than psychological response to cancer influence survival.

## EVERYONE IS AN INDIVIDUAL

While the dimensions of psychological distress will vary from patient to patient, emotional distress such as anxiety, sadness, or depression presents itself in different ways.

> The experience of chemotherapy is a nightmare! Losing control of your bodily functions, extreme nausea, no energy, made me suddenly feel hopeless.—Marsha, age 59. Breast cancer survivor.

Many cancer patients feel overwhelmed and are unable to get tasks done. Some report that they lack energy and have no motivation. Others report being unable to concentrate and feel that they are tired all the time. There is a sense of a loss of control. Some will cry a lot. While these manifestations can be characteristic of depression, it is important to distinguish depression from sadness. Depression is much more than feeling sad; there is a deep sense of hopelessness that the person with depression sees as permanent.

> When I was first told that I had breast cancer, many thoughts went through my mind: It can't be true. It can't be happening to me. I feel fine. They must be mistaken. I'm going to die.—Marsha, age 59. Breast cancer survivor.

Since a diagnosis of cancer is a major stressful event and since life, from then on, will never be the way it was before the diagnosis, the expression of sadness or distress could be considered to be a "normal" reaction to the diagnosis. These symptoms also can be triggered by the biological changes associated with cancer and its treatment. Many cancer medications cause psychological side effects, such as mood swings, and can bring on depression because of the effect they have on the body's chemistry. An alert medical team should be ready to provide those in need with appropriate care and counseling when "normal" distress elevates to abnormal levels of distress (severe anxiety, phobias, panic attacks, major depression). There are many options that can help individuals cope with the potentially debilitating side effects of cancer care. These include antidepressant medications, psychological counseling/therapy, and support groups.

Those newly diagnosed with breast cancer have to confront complex and difficult decisions about treatment. What may be appropriate for one woman may not be for another. The type of surgery and postoperative

## Table 9.1
## Psychosocial Model of Support

| | |
|---|---|
| *Feelings of Reassurance* | *Sense of Control* |
| Knowing what to expect | Able to make choices and decisions |
| Acceptance by family, friends | Information made available of disease |
| Support network | Information tailored to individual |
| *Organization of Care* | *Validation of Experience* |
| Integrated medical and psychological care | Being taken seriously |
| Continuity of care from diagnosis to remission | Acceptance of changes in appearance, lifestyle |
| Support for family | |

*Source:* Marlow, B, et al. An Interactive Process Model of Psychosocial Support Needs for Women Living with Breast Cancer. Psycho-oncology 12:319–30. 2003. p. 326.

treatment should be tailored to provide the most appropriate therapeutic care to the individual woman. As such, each individual needs to understand her options in order to make informed decisions. Butow and her colleagues have shown that the most sensitive and practical way of assessing psychosocial needs is to address each patient's needs according to individual coping style and circumstance.[10] A combination of specific types of psychosocial support matched to specific types of stress should offer the most effective level of support. As discussed in chapter 8, some individuals want as much information as possible to help them make decisions; others are content to defer to the physician. Some individuals can reach a decision somewhat quickly while others need time to consider and reflect on their options.

Marlow and her colleagues categorized psychosocial needs to reflect individual differences as well as needs at different stages of treatment and care. The categories are broad and highly interrelated to accommodate individual needs and styles of adjustment (table 9.1).[11]

## Organization of Care

Cancer patients express the importance of having access to an integrated information and support network from the time of diagnosis. There needs to be continuity of care throughout treatment and remission. The patient needs to know what to expect at each stage of treatment; for example, chemotherapy and radiotherapy often leave patients feeling worse than before the diagnosis of cancer was made.

## Sense of Control

After the initial shock of diagnosis, and the typically short period of time between diagnosis and treatment, many cancer patients express a sense of loss of control. Most cancer patients crave information about and involvement in decisions about treatment in order to gain some sense of control over their illness. When the individual can participate, to the desired degree, in a discussion about treatment alternatives, a sense of control is enhanced.

## Feeling of Reassurance

Cancer patients want to know what to expect in terms of their disease, their treatment, and prognosis. Patients want to be informed about not just the clinical aspects of their care but also the psychological effects of the disease. Acceptance by family and friends is mentioned by many cancer patients and reflects the need to be recognized as a person, not just as a cancer patient. Many individuals feel alienated from others; therefore, having a strong support network is critically important. Support groups provide a crucial source of reassurance.

## Validation of Experience

Breast cancer surgery may not be as major an operation as open heart surgery, but to the individual cancer patient, the ramifications are tremendous. A cancer patient wants to feel that family, friends, and the medical practitioners taking care of her understand her concerns and thoughts. A support network is a valuable means for cancer survivors to discuss their feelings, to be reassured by others who have experienced similar treatment, to adjust to their new realities of life.

## THE IMPORTANCE OF SUPPORT

Much has been written about the value of support networks. In particular, during the clinical course of the disease and its treatment, the presence of a strong social network can do much to help the individual cope. The importance of psychosocial support (informational and emotional) during and after cancer treatment is an important aspect of the care and recovery process.

Regardless of age, cancer patients often express that support from their husband or partner is a crucial element in coping. Those studies that have looked at this issue have found that, in general, patients who are older and who had better social support networks report less anxiety, and those who are older, married, had a higher educational level, or who had more social support report fewer depressive symptoms. Being married or living with a partner is associated with better general emotional health among a sample of women with breast cancer.[12]

Support comes in many forms: organized group support, individual support, Internet support groups, and support volunteer of the same age who underwent the same treatment. Support networks, organized by disease site, stage, and gender, are widely available for patients with cancer.

> What helped me the most is that I was given the names of others who were willing to speak to new patients. My "chemo pal" told me what to expect with the chemotherapy treatments to come. During radiation treatments, the patients all spoke about their particular problems. Everyone was very supportive and helpful. It really does help to talk about what is happening to you during such a stressful time.—Marsha, age 59. Breast cancer survivor.

Support networks, in whatever form, serve as an important source of comfort and offer a sense of reassurance; for example, learning what to expect from treatment or being told that one's emotions/feelings are normal. The effectiveness of support groups can vary depending on the individual's comfort in disclosing feelings and concerns as well as the perceived benefit of participating in a group. Among those who disclose, there is evidence to show that women more readily confide to their spouse, relatives, or friends more than they do to mental health workers. Women who tend not to disclose thoughts and feelings are more likely not to have strong social support networks or have unsupportive social interactions.[13]

Do support networks affect survival rates? Some studies have shown that group sessions for breast cancer had a positive effect on survival while others did not show a survival advantage. Some show a reduction in distress and a better quality of life. A large meta-analysis did not show a survival benefit across a number of interventions, although improvement of quality of life was apparent.[14]

## BREAST CANCER AND QUALITY OF LIFE ISSUES

In recent years, there has been more emphasis focused on understanding how being diagnosed and living with cancer affects an individual's quality of life. Quality of life is often measured as a subjective assessment of health status and well-being that include physical, psychological, social, and spiritual components. One study looked at psychosocial and demographic predictors of quality of life among a sample of 351 cancer patients asked to complete a series of self-report questionnaires assessing their social support, depression, anxiety, and quality of life. Findings show that patients who were older and had better social support reported less anxiety, and patients who were older, married, or who had more social support reported less depressive symptoms. Those who were older, married, with more formal education, less advanced disease, and better social support reported better quality of life in the mental health domain, independent of demographic and medical variables.[15]

An interesting finding of this study is that despite the fact that many patients reported significant depressive symptoms, they reported generally good quality of life in the mental health domain. This suggests that although patients have some symptoms of distress, overall they consider their functioning to be reasonably good. They believe that they are functioning well considering their current health condition. While this study identified several predictors of quality of life and psychological adjustment, which had been found in other studies, it highlighted the importance of evaluating individual patient characteristics and psychosocial factors in patients with cancer.

Since an increasing number of women are surviving for years after their diagnosis, issues such as body image, relationships, financial or vocational issues, and sexual relations are reported as being particularly important to address. Issues relating to sexuality, reestablishment of intimacy, and concerns about dating may seem trivial during the early phases of treatment, but become hugely important after completion of treatment. Removal of all or part of the breast, hair loss, weight gain, reduction in libido, and sexual dysfunction secondary to estrogen problems can impact sexual relations regardless of the age of the survivor. But, the long-term reproductive impact of breast cancer treatment uniquely affects the younger, premenopausal breast cancer survivor.

Understanding the issues related to premature menopause and fertility among breast cancer survivors, and patients' information needs about these issues, is especially important in light of the fact that more women are delaying childbearing.[16] Chemotherapy, in particular, carries with it reproductive and gynecological implications that younger women may find complicate plans for childbearing. In addition, due to the rapid change in menopausal status in chemotherapy-induced ovarian failure, the symptoms of menopause can be more severe than those that occur with natural aging.[17]

Early menopause may also have an adverse impact on sexual functioning. A large study of breast cancer survivors found that younger women and those with treatment-induced menopause are more likely to experience sexual dysfunction following treatment for breast cancer.[18] Discussion of fertility and menopause at the time of diagnosis is probably more than a young woman can handle. The shock of the diagnosis and the fear of mortality probably overshadow any comprehension of a discussion of their fertility-related information needs. While some physicians may address fertility issues before treatment, others prefer to discuss fertility and menopause-related information during or following treatment for breast cancer, or around the time that a patient might consider becoming pregnant.

## REGAINING A SENSE OF CONTROL

Over the past decades, it has been shown that information, counseling, and supportive care can increase overall well-being in women with breast cancer. While the evidence is mixed regarding whether they have any substantial affect on survival, it is clearer that feelings of well-being, reassurance, and a sense of control can be improved. Many women have said that their sense of control is enhanced when they have information relevant to themselves. Unfortunately, while supportive care interventions are valuable, many women are not referred to such programs. Given that there is evidence that such interventions are helpful, if real gains in the well-being of women with breast cancer are to be made, there must be a greater, more concerted effort to routinely include supportive care programs in the treatment process.[19]

Since an overwhelming majority of women are surviving for years after being diagnosed with breast cancer, the psychological issues facing breast cancer survivors are increasingly important to acknowledge and address. For the young breast cancer patients, especially those who have young children, concerns have been expressed about not only the ability to cope with family responsibilities as well as the disease, but also what effect their diagnosis of cancer will have on the children. Financial concerns are expressed by both older and younger women with breast cancer. Loss of income and/or loss of job due to cancer treatment are significant worries for both groups.

Many organizations have programs available to help cancer patients and survivors. Social workers, part of the care-giving team, can provide education, counseling, and referrals to community or national agencies and support groups. Psychological counseling, either individually or in a group, is another option to help patients and their families discuss issues of concern, develop and enhance coping strategies, help the individual regain a sense of control over her life, and improve her quality of life. Mental health providers can create a treatment plan to meet a patient's specific needs. Financial counseling might be needed, and a financial counselor is well equipped to answer questions about financial issues related to medical care.

Information, emotional support, and help in decision making are available both from support groups as well as from Internet-based systems of integrated services. Face-to-face support groups are useful for sharing experiences and information. Support groups can be either peer led or professionally led and can be time limited or open ended. The American Cancer Society's Reach to Recovery program, for example, for more than thirty years has been helping breast cancer patients cope with their disease. Through face-to-face visits or by phone, specially trained volunteers offer understanding, support, and hope. The CHESS system, developed at the University of Wisconsin, is an example of a computer-based system that provides information, social support, decision-making and problem-solving tools in one easy-to-use system. It tailors and personalizes information, protects privacy, and details health information in several languages. Appendix A provides a listing of Web sites and organizations that provide support to cancer patients.

## HOW HEALTH-CARE PROVIDERS CAN
## MAKE A DIFFERENCE

Numerous studies have shown that how and to what extent the physician responds to the patient's emotional needs is very important. That is, the physician's sensitive response to a patient's emotional distress reduces or ameliorates psychological distress.[20] A clearly explained, individually tailored delivery of information by the physician can do much to help allay patient fears and anxiety.[21] Implicit in this, however, is that the physician is able to discern and detect a patient's needs for information and emotional support. Unfortunately, physicians, more often than not, fail to elicit their patients' emotional and informational concerns.

Physicians, in particular, are generally deficient in detecting patients' emotional needs.[22] Many physicians are far more comfortable dealing with the clinical aspects of their patients' care as well as meeting the direct informational needs of their patients than they are in dealing with the emotional and psychological issues that certainly accompany cancer care.[23] While most physicians are able to respond to a patient's direct expressions of need, they have greater difficulty in detecting and responding to indirect or nonverbal patient cues such as facial expression, posture, or tone of voice. Yet, listening to the patient and being receptive to verbal and nonverbal cues can alert the health-care provider to a patient's psychological needs.

Of course the extent and severity of psychological symptoms will vary greatly among patients, but it is rare that a patient would not suffer some psychological fallout from her disease. Perhaps complicating the issue is that not every patient feels comfortable disclosing or discussing her emotional problems directly to her health-care team. Some perceive doctors as busy people who maybe should not be burdened with the patient's worries or fears. For others, they may feel that their worries are "normal" under the circumstances; therefore, the doctor should not be "bothered" with such problems. Those with a more fatalistic attitude may feel that an emotional response to their cancer is reflective of their belief that nothing can be done about it anyway and are reluctant to share their feelings. Among those who do not want to be seen as uncooperative or ungrateful, these individuals might be more likely to allude indirectly to their emotional needs rather than to directly express their feelings. Given that there are different ways of expressing emotion, it is important that the medical team be astute to pick up on nonverbal cues such as body language and body posture, and to reach out to those patients who are unable to express their emotional concerns directly.

Patient and physician behavior, then, are associated with how well a patient's emotional needs are detected and addressed. To some extent, the onus necessarily falls on the physician to encourage the patient to talk about her emotional needs, no matter how trivial. Being attentive to facial expressions, posture and other indirect clues can help the physician raise the issue of emotional need. Gentle but direct questioning of emotional status should be included as part of the consultation. Showing empathy, too, can signal the patient that the physician is concerned and cares about her. When the physician responds in this manner, the patient should perceive that talking about her emotional state is welcome and important.

Patient interactions with others, particularly with the nurses or with the clergy, often will provide with emotional support needed. The nurse is a pivotal person as this individual is usually the one to find out how distressed the patient is and what kind of problems she is having. Patients are generally more open and willing to unburden themselves to a nurse or clergy rather than to the physician. Both nurses and clergy are good, compassionate listeners and can make recommendations on a range of interventions from spiritual counseling to various kinds of psychotherapy.

## FEAR OF RECURRENCE

> What stays in my mind is always the question: Will I get it back? When??? I am a high risk cancer survivor, so I am well aware that this is a strong possibility. I suppose that this will always be with me.—Marsha, age 59. Cancer survivor.

The end of treatment marks a time of psychosocial adjustment to recovery. There will be constant reminders of the disease that could trigger psychological crises: anniversary dates, follow-up checkups, and the like. Probably the greatest threat to psychological well-being is coping with recurrence and/or advanced, end-stage disease. There are three types of recurrent breast cancer: local (cancerous tumor cells remain in the original site and over time grow back), regional (the cancer has spread past the site), and distant (the cancer has metastasized to other parts of the body). A recurrence of noninvasive breast cancer is far less serious than a recurrence of invasive cancer. Breast cancer has the potential to spread to almost any region of the body although the most common sites include the bone, lung, brain, or liver. Distant recurrence of breast cancer is very serious, and the survival rate is considerably lower than for women whose cancer is confined to the breast or axillary lymph nodes. Besides local and regional recurrences, a new cancer may occasionally occur years after the initial cancer.

Often a diagnosis of recurrent cancer is more devastating or psychologically difficult for a woman than her initial breast cancer diagnosis. Patients with recurrence have fears and concerns different from those at first diagnosis; feelings of injustice, discouragement, hopelessness are commonly cited. The emotional roller coaster of coping with the recurrence, as well as the recognition of one's mortality, is hugely stressful for the patient and her family. My mother felt betrayed when, fifteen years after her initial battle with breast cancer, she was diagnosed with advanced, distant recurrence. The fear of her own mortality, the anger of having to undergo radiation and chemotherapy again, the injustice of it all, made her furious. But, she never gave up her fight until three months before her death, when the rapidly spreading cancer finally sapped her will to live.

## WHAT IS PSYCHO-ONCOLOGY?

Recognizing the importance of and need for psychological support during and after cancer treatment, the medical profession understood the value of developing a specialty area that would deal with the myriad of neuropsychiatric and psychological issues stemming from cancer therapies. As medical care is increasingly delivered outside of the hospital, the burden on families became significant. Fatigue, mood and cognitive problems, incontinence, impotence, chronic pain syndromes, and peripheral neuropathy are common complications of some chemotherapy treatments. The need for psychiatric/psychological support is particularly important to help the patient and the family cope.

The subspecialty of psycho-oncology began formally in the mid-1970s, around the same time that the stigma of revealing the diagnosis of cancer faded, making it more acceptable to talk with a patient about the disease and the implications for her life. Psycho-oncology focuses on the social, behavioral, and ethical aspects of cancer. It addresses the psychological responses of patients to cancer at all stages of the disease, as well as that of their families and the providers of care. It is a multidisciplinary field that includes surgery, medicine, oncology, pediatrics, radiotherapy, epidemiology, immunology, endocrinology, pathology, bioethics, and psychiatry. Working collaboratively, the object is to assess and treat psychological reactions at all stages of the cancer as well as the stresses on the family and the clinical staff.[24]

In an effort to set standards for this new discipline, the National Comprehensive Cancer Network, an organization of eighteen comprehensive cancer centers, established a multidisciplinary panel to develop standards for psychosocial care in cancer. These standards, based on those developed for pain, require that all patients be evaluated initially and monitored for the level and nature of their psychosocial distress (a term that was deemed to be less stigmatizing than other psychological terms). Distress encompasses a range from normal feelings of vulnerability, sadness, and fear to more disabling conditions such as clinical depression, anxiety, panic, isolation, and spiritual crisis.[25]

## END NOTE

Breast cancer has shifted from being seen as a largely fatal illness to one that is a chronic disease. The majority of those diagnosed will live for years after their treatment. As such, the psychosocial correlates of breast cancer are now seen to be as important as the medical treatment of the disease. The provision of optimal care requires the use of a multidisciplinary team that, importantly, includes mental health professionals and makes use of support networks. The diagnosis and treatment of breast cancer is a stressful time for both the patient and her family. In addition to the physical changes that accompany breast cancer, changes in behavior and mood are very common. For those suffering from common stress signals such as disturbed sleep, fatigue, pain, anxiety, and irritability, or depression, help should be sought or offered by those close to the individual. Regaining a sense of control may take time, but with the help of the medical team and family and friends, a sense of control and confidence can be achieved.

# The Breast Self-Exam

Breast self-exams (BSE) are useful to help detect changes in the breast. Since the common symptoms of breast cancer include lumps, dimpling, or thickening of the breast tissue and nipple discharge, a BSE can help a woman monitor how her breasts normally look and feel. Since many breast lumps are found by women themselves, the purpose of a monthly BSE is to note any abnormalities in the breast or nipple. While most breast lumps are not cancerous, a physician should perform a clinical breast exam to rule out serious disease. Delaying the diagnosis of breast cancer does not change the diagnosis, but it could worsen the outcome.

## WHEN TO DO A BSE

BSEs should be done monthly, two to three days after menstruation stops. For those women who are in menopause, picking one day (the first of the month, for example) to do a BSE is suggested.

## HOW TO DO A BSE

Lie on your back and flatten the right breast by placing a pillow under your right shoulder. Then place your right arm behind your head. Using the middle three fingers of your left hand in a circular motion feel for lumps around the breast. One should press lightly at first without probing the breast tissue. Then, apply medium pressure, pressing midway into the breast tissue. Finally, press firmly enough to probe more deeply.

You should completely feel all of the breast and chest area up to and under the armpit and up to the collarbone and over to the shoulder. Another procedure is to start in the underarm area and move your fingers downward until below the breast. Continue until the entire breast has been probed. Or, you could begin at the outer edge of the breast and move around the breast in concentric circles until the entire breast has been palpated.

Whichever method you choose, repeat the process on the left breast by placing a pillow under the left shoulder and using the right hand to examine the left breast.

A BSE can be done while standing in the shower when the skin is soapy. In this case, raise one arm behind your head and use the opposite hand to examine the opposite breast in the same manner as just described.

Check both breasts for changes in texture and shape by looking in a mirror. A physician should investigate any dimpling of the skin or nipple discharge.

# Listing of Types of Support Groups/Organizations

There are thousands of breast cancer–related groups, organizations, and information on the Internet, and finding the appropriate information can be overwhelming. The following is provided merely as a reference. It is not a comprehensive listing by any means.

Web Sites:

http://www.cancerindex.org/clinks is a guide to Internet resources for cancer. It provides over 4,000 links to cancer related information and resources including telephone help lines, patient guides, and resources for caregivers. It is regularly updated.

http://www.cancer.org/docroot/ESN/content links to the American Cancer Society's Reach to Recovery program. Through face-to-face visits or by phone Reach to Recovery volunteers provide support and up-to-date information.

http://www.breastcancer.org is a Web site that specializes in providing information and support to help women cope with breast cancer.

http://www.cancerhopenetwork.org provides free and confidential one-on-one support to cancer patients and their families utilizing trained volunteers who have undergone and recovered from a similar cancer experience.

http://www.insuranceforsurvivors.com specializes in insurance for cancer survivors.

http://www.lbbc.org is a nonprofit educational organization whose purpose is to focus on the physical, social, emotional, legal, and financial issues women face after completing breast cancer treatment. The Web site maintains several breast cancer message boards designed to bring women with breast cancer together.

http://www.lookgoodfeelbetter.org is a free, national public service program that provides information about beauty techniques to help women adjust to their appearance and self-image during and after treatment.

http://www.breast-cancer-support.com provides a venue for patients and survivors to share their experiences about all aspects of breast cancer.

http://www.oncochat.org is a Web chat site and also maintains an extensive directory of online resources related to cancer support, treatment, and research.

http://www.onepinkribbon.com is a Web site focusing on personal strategies to help patients cope with their cancer diagnosis and treatment. The focus is on coaching, a form of therapy that emphasizes personal strategies to help patients cope.

http://www.imaginis.com/breasthealth/breast_protheses.asp lists companies that manufacture breast prostheses.

http://www.imaginis.com/breasthealth/hair_loss.asp lists companies that provide hair loss accessories.

http://www.cancer.org/tlc/turbans.html is sponsored by the American Cancer Society and offers a variety of accessories for those who have experienced hair loss.

http://www.wellness-community.org helps cancer patients and their families by providing a professional program of emotional support, education, and hope.

http://www.nabco.org (National Alliance of Breast Cancer Organizations) is a membership and advocacy organization of over 300 breast cancer organizations that provides individualized information package on breast cancer treatment, support services, and financial assistance. It produces a listing of national resources including printed materials, videos, hotlines, and a database of support organizations.

http://www.y-me.org provides presurgical information and referral and phone counseling. Hotline volunteers are breast cancer survivors.

# Additional Resources Regarding Clinical Trials

The importance of the randomized double-blinded clinical trial is discussed in the chapters of this book. In essence, the randomized controlled clinical trial is the best way to conclusively determine whether a new treatment is better than a placebo, or whether a new drug is better than the one currently prescribed. Despite the importance of the clinical trial, it can be difficult to enroll patients. Not every patient is an appropriate subject as every trial has an inclusion and exclusion criteria. By virtue of the randomization process, a group of participants will not receive the drug or treatment, but will be given a placebo or the non-experimental drug. Those enrolling in a trial hoping to receive the experimental drug, for example, may be quite disappointed to learn how trials are run. In other cases, the burdens of participating in the trial may be too much, prompting some to drop out before the end of the study; for example, maybe the side effects of the treatment were too uncomfortable or maybe the need for repeated testing was too burdensome.

Physicians, too, must determine whether the trial is potentially beneficial to a patient. That is, the risks must not outweigh the benefits. Physicians must feel comfortable referring patients and must be able to explain the risks and the benefits to the patient. He or she must have the ability to introduce and sufficiently explain the nature of the clinical trial so that the patient can make an informed decision.

For those patients who are so inclined, there are numerous online clinical trial listings for specific diseases. Each site has a searchable database and provides descriptions of trials. The following gives some examples of commonly referred to Web sites:

| Web Site | Affiliation |
| --- | --- |
| www.clinical_trials.gov | National Institutes of Health |
| www.cancer.gov/clinicaltrials | National Cancer Institute |
| www.clinicaltrials.cancer.org | American Cancer Society |
| www.clinicaltrials.com | Pharmaceutical Research Plus, Inc. |
| www.veritasmedicine.com | Private corporation |
| www.centerwatch.com | Private corporation |

Those considering clinical trials also could obtain a copy of the National Cancer Institute's booklet, *Taking Part in Clinical Trials: What Cancer Patients Need to Know*. This booklet describes how research trials are carried out and explains the risks and the benefits. The booklet can be obtained from http://cancer.gov/publications.

# Additional Resources and References Regarding Mammography

The FDA Web site (http://www.fda.gov/cdrh/mammography) publishes reports on the performance of mammography facilities based on the Mammography Quality Standards Act (MQSA) inspection. These reports list adverse events including the revocation of medical licenses or actions taken against a mammography facility, including the reason for the action, corrective actions, and status of the facility.

The FDA Mammography Site Database is useful to search for the location of mammography facilities: http://www.accessdata.fda.gov/scripts/cdrh/cfdocs/cfmqsa/search.cfm.

# Glossary

**Adjuvant Therapy:**   a cancer treatment method used in addition to (adjuvant to) surgery, radiation, chemotherapy, or hormone therapy.

**Allele:**   any one of a series of two or more different genes that may occupy the same position or locus on a specific chromosome.

**Axillary Lymph Node Dissection:**   surgery to remove some of the lymph nodes in the armpit.

**Axillary Node:**   one of the lymph glands of the axilla (armpit) that help to fight infections in the chest, armpit, neck, and arm and to drain lymph from those areas.

**Benign:**   noncancerous growth.

**Biopsy:**   the removal and microscopic examination of tissue for diagnosis. A biopsy can be done surgically or with needles.

**BRCA1:**   a gene, when mutated, that increases the risk of breast or ovarian cancer, or both.

**BRCA2:**   a gene, when mutated, that increases the risk of breast cancer.

**Breast-Conserving Surgery:**   surgery that removes only the tumor and a small amount of surrounding breast tissue. (Example: lumpectomy).

**Breast Self-Exam:**   physical examination of the breasts by the woman with the intent of finding lumps or other unusual signs of breast disease.

**Cancer:**   a group of diseases in which cells are changed in appearance and function, grow out of control, and form a mass (tumor) that can spread to surrounding tissues or organs.

**Chemotherapy:**   cancer treatment by means of chemical substances or drugs designed to kill or damage cancer cells.

**Clinical Breast Exam:**   physical examination of the breasts by a physician or trained health professional with the intent of finding lumps or other unusual signs of breast disease.

**Clinical Outcome:**   end result of a medical intervention (e.g., survival, improved health, death).

**Clinical Trial:**   a study intended to quantify the safety or effectiveness of a drug, a procedure, or a medical intervention. Clinical trials can be randomized or not randomized.

**Computer-Aided Detection:**   the use of sophisticated computer programs designed to recognize patterns in images.

**Detection:**   finding disease. Early detection means that the disease is found at an early, more treatable, stage.

**Diagnosis:**   confirmation of a disease usually as a result of laboratory findings or radiological imaging.

**Diagnostic Mammography:**   X-ray-based breast imaging. The purpose is to diagnose an abnormality discovered by physical exam or screening mammography.

**Digital Mammography:**   type of mammogram.

**Duct:**   a hollow passage for gland secretions. In the breast, it is a passage through which milk passes from the lobule to the nipple.

**Ductal Carcinoma In Situ (DCIS):**   a lesion consisting of abnormal cells within the ducts of the breast, but with no viable evidence of invasion into the duct walls or the surrounding tissues. Sometimes DCIS is referred to as precancer or preinvasive cancer.

**Ductal Lavage:**   a procedure in which a small catheter is inserted into the breast nipple and the breast ducts are flushed with fluid to collect breast cells.

**Dysplasia:**   abnormal change in cells leading to abnormal growth. Cells in the tissue do not look normal. (Compare to hyperplasia).

**Effectiveness:**   the extent to which a specific test or intervention does what it is intended to do.

**Epidemiology:**   the science of quantifying the distribution and determinants of disease in populations.

**Excisional Biopsy:**   surgery that completely removes a small breast lump during tissue sampling for examination under the microscope to see if cancer cells are present. This is not a lumpectomy.

**False Negative:**   a test result that indicates an abnormality or disease is not present when in fact it is.

**False Positive:**   a test result that indicates an abnormality or disease is present when in fact it is not.

**Fine-Needle Aspiration:**   a procedure by which a thin needle is used to collect fluid and/or cells from a breast lump for microscopic examination.

**Hormone Therapy:**   cancer treatment in which drugs are used to slow tumor growth by blocking the effect of certain hormones. Designed to prevent cancer recurrence.

**Hormones:**   substances made by the body that regulate the activity of certain cells or organs.

**Hyperplasia:**   an increase in the number of cells. Altered cells divide in an uncontrolled manner leading to an excess of cells in tissue. Cells have a normal appearance, but there are too many of them.

**Incidence:**   the number of new cases of a disease in a study population at a specific time period.

**Invasive Cancer:**   cancerous tumors that have grown beyond their site of origin and have invaded surrounding tissue.

**Invasive Ductal Carcinoma:**   a cancer that originates in the ducts of the breast and breaks through the duct wall to invade the surrounding tissue. It is the most common type of breast cancer, accounting for 80 percent of breast malignancies.

**Invasive Lobular Carcinoma:**   a cancer that originates in the milk-producing glands (lobules) of the breast to invade surrounding tissue. This type of breast cancer accounts for 15 percent of invasive breast cancers.

**Lobular Carcinoma In Situ:**   abnormal cells within a breast lobule but that have not invaded surrounding tissue.

**Lump:**   any kind of mass in the breast or other parts of the body.

**Lumpectomy:**   the partial surgical removal of tissue from the breast.

**Lymphedema:**   swelling of the arm caused by malfunctioning lymphatic drainage. Occurs on the side of the body where the mastectomy or axillary dissection was performed.

**Lymph Nodes:**   part of the lymphatic system that helps fight infection.

**Magnetic Resonance Imaging (MRI):**   a radiologic method by which images are created. It is designed to show tumors before they can be felt.

**Malignancy:**   a cancerous tumor that tends to spread to surrounding tissues or organs.

**Mammogram:**   X-ray image of the breast. It is designed to show tumors in the breast before they can be felt.

**Mastectomy:**   surgical removal of the breast.

**Metastasis:**   spread of a cancer from one part of the body to another. Cells in the new cancer are the same cell type as the original cancer.

**Microcalcifications:**  tiny calcium deposits within the breast. They are often found by mammography and may be a sign of cancer.

**Modified Radical Mastectomy:**  surgery that removes the entire breast including some axillary lymph nodes.

**Molecular Markers:**  changes in cells at the molecular level. These changes may be indicative of potential cancer.

**Mutation:**  a change in the character of a gene that is perpetuated in subsequent divisions of the cell in which it occurs.

**Oncogene:**  the gene that contributes to the development of a malignant tumor.

**Oncologist:**  a physician who specializes in the treatment of cancers.

**Palpable Tumor:**  a tumor that can be felt by hand.

**Partial Mastectomy:**  surgical removal of part of the breast.

**Population-Based Survey:**  a survey conducted to estimate the prevalence of a disease in a population.

**Positron Emission Tomography (PET):**  use of radioactive tracers to identify regions in the body with altered metabolic activity.

**Premalignant:**  changes in cells that may precede the development of a malignant tumor. Also called precancer.

**Prevalence:**  number of existing cases of disease in a population at a specified time period.

**Prognosis:**  prediction of the course and end of disease and the estimated chance for recovery.

**Psycho-Oncology:**  an area in medicine that focuses on the social, behavioral, and ethnical aspects of cancer care for the patient, family, and providers of care.

**Radiation Therapy:**  treatment for breast cancer that uses high-energy rays to destroy cancer.

**Randomized Clinical Trials:**  patients are enrolled in a study (for example, comparing a treatment or drug to a placebo) and randomly assigned to the treatment group or the control group.

**Recurrence:**  reappearance of the cancer. Recurrence can be local (at the same site), regional (near the original site), or distant (in another site).

**Scintimammography:**  use of radioactive tracers to produce an image of the breast.

**Screening:**  examination of an asymptomatic sample of a population with the goal to detect a specific disease at an early stage.

**Screening Mammography:**  X-ray-based breast imaging in an asymptomatic population with the goal to detect breast tumors at an early stage.

**Selective Estrogen Receptor Modulators (SERMs):**  agents that function as estrogen agonists in the tissues in which estrogen is beneficial but that will function as estrogen antagonists in sites where estrogen may promote carcinogenesis. Tamoxifen and raloxifene are examples for SERMs.

**Sensitivity:**   the proportion of truly diseased persons in a screened population who are identified as diseased by the screening test (true positive rate).

**Specificity:**   the proportion of truly nondiseased persons who are so identified by the screening test (true negative rate).

**Tamoxifen:**   hormonal drug that blocks estrogen.

**Total Mastectomy:**   surgery to remove the entire breast but not the axillary lymph nodes or muscular tissue beneath the breast. Also known as simple mastectomy.

**Tumor:**   an abnormal mass of tissue that results from excessive cell division. Tumors can be benign or malignant.

**Tumor Marker:**   any substance or characteristic that indicates the presence of a malignancy.

**Ultrasound:**   inaudible, high-frequency sound waves used to create an image of the body.

# Notes

Literally thousands of articles have been published on the topic. The following is a selective list of references. Use of secondary sources such as textbooks, reviews, commentaries, and Web sites is made to limit the list of references. The reader is encouraged to consult Web sites listed at the end of each chapter for further information.

## CHAPTER 1

1. Yalom, M. A History of the Breast. New York: Alfred A. Knopf. 1998.
2. History of the Bra. bformfaq@blooberry.com.
3. History of the Bra, or Brassiere. PageWise, Inc. 2001.
4. Cancer Reference Information. http://www.cancer.org.
5. Diseases of the Breast. http://www.mayoclinic.com.
6. Li, CI, Anderson, BO, Daling, JR, et al. Trends in Incidence Rates of Invasive Lobular and Ductal Breast Carcinoma. Journal of the American Medical Association 289:1421–224. 2003.
7. Li, CI, Weiss, NS, Stanford, JL, et al. Hormone Replacement Therapy in Relation to the Risk of Lobular and Ductal Breast Carcinoma in Middle-aged Women. Cancer 88:2570–77. 2000; Chen, CL, Weiss, NS, Newcomb, P, et al. Hormone Replacement Therapy in Relation to Breast Cancer. Journal of the American Medical Association 287:734–41. 2002; Newcomb, PA, Titus-Ermstoff, L, Egan, KM, et al. Post-menopausal Estrogen

and Progestin Use in Relation to Breast Cancer Risk. Cancer Epidemiology, Biomarkers and Prevention 11:593–600. 2002; Daling, JR, Malone, KE, Doody, DR, et al. Relation of Regimens of Combined Hormone Replacement Therapy to Lobular, Ductal, and other Histologic Types of Breast Carcinoma. Cancer 95:2455–64. 2002.

8. Harris, JR, Lippman, ME, Morrow, M, Osborne, CK. Diseases of the Breast. Philadelphia: Lippincott Williams and Wilkins. 2000.

9. Burstein, HJ, Polyak, K, Wong, JS, et al. Ductal Carcinoma in Situ of the Breast. New England Journal of Medicine 350:1430–41. 2004.

10. Ernster, VL, Ballard-Barbash, R, Barlow, WE, et al. Detection of Ductal Carcinoma in Situ in Women Undergoing Screening Mammography. Journal of the National Cancer Institute 94:1546–54. 2002.

11. Claus, EB, Stowe, M, Carter, D. Breast Carcinoma in Situ: Risk Factors and Screening Patterns. Journal of the National Cancer Institute 93:1811–17. 2001.

12. Ernster, VL, Barclay, J, Kerlikowske, K, et al. Mortality Among Women with Ductal Carcinoma in Situ of the Breast in the Population-Based Surveillance, Epidemiology and End Results Program. Archives of Internal Medicine 160:953–58. 2000.

13. Cutuli, B, Lemanski, C, LeBlanc, M, et al. Local Recurrences after DCIS Therapy: Diagnosis, Treatment, Outcome. Breast Cancer Research and Treatment 76: Suppl1:536. Abstract. 2002.

## CHAPTER 2

1. Cancer Facts and Figures. American Cancer Society. 2003.

2. Giordano, SH, Cohen, DS, Buzdar, AM, et al. Breast Carcinoma in Men. Cancer 101:51–57. 2004.

3. Cancer Facts and Figures. Op cit.

4. Feuer, EJ, Wun, LM. DEVCAN: Probability of Developing or Dying of Cancer. Version 4.0. Bethesda, MD: National Cancer Institute. 1999.

5. Morris, CR, Wright, WE, Schlag, ED. The Risk of Developing Breast Cancer within the Next 5, 10, or 20 Years of a Woman's Life. American Journal of Preventive Medicine 20:214–18. 2001.

6. Ursin, G, Spicer, DV, Bernstein, L. Breast Cancer Epidemiology, Treatment, and Prevention. In Goldman, MB and Hatch, MC (eds). Women and Health. New York: Academic Press. 2000. pp. 871–83.

7. Ibid.

8. Li, CI, Malone, KE, Daling, JR. Differences in Breast Cancer Stage, Treatment, and Survival by Race and Ethnicity. Archives of Internal Medicine 163:49–56. 2003.

9. Bradley, CJ, Given, CW, Roberts, C. Race, Socioeconomic Status, and Breast Cancer Treatment and Survival. Journal of the National Cancer Institute 94:490–96. 2002.

10. Newman, B. Inherited Genetic Susceptibility and Breast Cancer. In Goldman, MB and Hatch, MC (eds). Women and Health. New York: Academic Press. 2000. pp. 884–94.

11. Scheuer, L, Kauff, N, Robson, M, et al. Outcome of Preventive Surgery and Screening for Breast and Ovarian Cancer in BRCA Mutation Carriers. Journal of Clinical Oncology Mar 1:1260–68. 2002.

12. King, MC, Marks, JH, Mandell, JB. Breast and Ovarian Cancer Risks Due to Inherited Mutations in BRCA1 and BRCA2. Science 302:643–46. 2003.

13. Ford, D, Easton, DF, Peto, J. Estimates of the Gene Frequency of BRCA1 and its Contribution to Breast and Ovarian Cancer Incidence. American Journal of Human Genetics 60:496–504. 1995.

14. King, MC, Marks, JH, Mandell, JB, et al. Breast and Ovarian Cancer Risks Due to Inherited Mutations in BRCA1 and BRCA2. Science 302:643–46. 2003.

15. Thurfjell, E. Breast Density and the Risk of Breast Cancer. New England Journal of Medicine 347:866. 2002.

16. Ursin, G, Spicer, DV, Bernstein, L. Breast Cancer Epidemiology, Treatment, and Prevention. In Goldman, MB and Hatch, MC. Women & Health. San Diego, CA: Academic Press. 2000. pp. 871–83.

17. Enger, SM, Ross, RK, Hnderson, B, et al. Breast Feeding History, Pregnancy Experience and Risk of Breast Cancer. British Journal of Cancer 76: 118–23. 1997; Enger, SM, Ross, RK, Paganini-Hill, A, et al. Breastfeeding Experience and Breast Cancer Risk Among Postmenopausal Women. Cancer Epidemiology, Biomarkers, and Prevention 7:365–69. 1998.

18. Calle, EE, Rodriguez, C, Walker-Thurmond, K, et al. Overweight, Obesity, and Mortality from Cancer in a Prospectively Studied Cohort of U.S. Adults. New England Journal of Medicine 348:1625–38. 2003.

19. Horn-Ross, PL, Hoggatt, KJ, West, DW, et al. Recent Diet and Breast Cancer Risk: The California Teachers Study (USA). Cancer Causes and Control 13:407–15. 2002; Webb, PM, Byrne, C, Schnitt, SJ, et al. A Prospective Study of Diet and Benign Breast Disease. Cancer Epidemiology, Biomarkers, and Prevention 13:1106–13. 2004; Holmes, MD, Willett, WC. Does Diet Affect Breast Cancer Risk? Breast Cancer Research 6:170–78. 2004.

20. Lee, MI. Physical Activity in Women: How Much is Good Enough? Journal of the American Medical Association 290:1377–79. 2003.

21. Vaino, H, Bianchini, R (eds). And the International Agency for Research on Cancer Working Group on the Evaluation of Cancer Preventive

Agents. Weight Control and Physical Activity. Lyon, France: International Agency for Research on Cancer. IARC Handbook on Cancer Prevention. Vol 6. 2002.

22. McTiernan, A, Kooperberg, C, White, E, et al. Recreational Physical Activity and the Risk of Breast Cancer in Postmenopausal Women. Journal of the American Medical Association 290:1331–36. 2003.

23. Gammon, MD, Neugut, AI, Santella, RM, et al. The Long Island Breast Cancer Study Project: Description of a Multi-institutional Collaboration to Identify Environmental Risk Factors for Breast Cancer. Breast Cancer Research and Treatment 74:235–54. 2002.

24. Ibid.

25. Collaborative Group on Hormonal Factors in Breast Cancer: Breast Cancer and Hormonal Contraceptives: Collaborative Reanalysis of Individual Data on 53,297 Women with Breast Cancer and 100,239 Women without Breast Cancer from 54 Epidemiological Studies. Lancet 347:1713–27. 1996.

26. Marchbanks, PA, McDonald, JA, Wilson, HG, et al. Oral Contraceptives and the Risk of Breast Cancer. New England Journal of Medicine 346: 2025–32. 2002.

27. Finkel, ML, Cohen, M, Mahoney, H. Treatment Options for the Menopausal Woman. Nurse Practitioner 26:5–15. 2001.

28. Collaborative Group on Hormonal Factors in Breast Cancer. Op cit.

29. Writing Group for the Women's Health Initiative Investigation. Risks and Benefits of Estrogen Plus Progestin in Healthy Postmenopausal Women: Principal Results for the Women's Health Initiative Randomized Clinical Trial. Journal of the American Medical Association 288:321–33. 2002; Fletcher, SW, Colditz, GA. Failure of Estrogen Plus Progestin Treatment for Prevention. Journal of the American Medical Association 288:366–68. 2002.

30. Chlebowski, RT, Hendrix, SL, Langer, RD, et al. Influence of Estrogen Plus Progestin on Breast Cancer and Mammography in Healthy Postmenopausal Women: The Women's Health Initiative Randomized Trial. Journal of the American Medical Association 289:3243–53. 2003.

31. Gann, P, Morrow, M. Combined Hormone Therapy and Breast Cancer. Journal of the American Medical Association 289:3304–6. 2003.

32. NIH Asks Participants in Women's Health Initiative Estrogen-Alone Study to Stop Study Pills. DHHS. NIH News. March 2, 2004.

33. Li, CI, Anderson, BO, Daling, JR, et al. Trends in Incident Rates of Invasive Lobular and Ductal Breast Carcinoma. Journal of the American Medical Association 289:1421–24. 2003.

34. Ghafoor, A, Hemal, A, Ward, E, et al. Trends in Breast Cancer by Race and Ethnicity. CA Cancer Journal for Clinicians 53:342–55. 2003.

35. Malone, KE. Diethylstilbestrol (DES) and Breast Cancer. Epidemiology Review 15:108–9.1993.
36. Smith-Warner, SA, Spiegelman, D, Yaun, SS, et al. Alcohol and Breast Cancer in Women: A Pooled Analysis of Cohort Studies. Journal of the American Medical Association 279:535–40. 1998.
37. Wingo, PA, Cardinez, CJ, Landis, SH, et al. Long-Term Trends in Cancer Mortality in the United States, 1930–1998. Cancer S97:3133–265. 2003.
38. Cancer Facts and Figures. American Cancer Society. 2003.
39. Health, United States: 2002. Mammography. Table 82. National Center for Health Statistics. http://www.cdc.gov/nchs.fastats/mammogram.html.
40. Li, CI, Malone, KE, Daling, JR. Op.cit.

## CHAPTER 3

1. Cancer Staging. http://www.cancerquest.org; Staging-Specific Patterns of Breast Cancer. http://oesi.nci.nih.gov.
2. Veronesi, V, Cascinelli, N, Mariani, L, et al. Twenty-year Follow Up of a Randomized Trial Comparing Total Mastectomy, Lumpectomy, and Lumpectomy Plus Irradiation for the Treatment of Invasive Breast Cancer. New England Journal of Medicine 347:1233–41. 2002.
3. Fisher, B, Anderson, S, Bryant, J, et al. Twenty-year Follow Up of a Randomized Study Comparing Beast-Conserving Surgery with Radical Mastectomy for Early Breast Cancer. New England Journal of Medicine 347:1227–32. 2002.
4. Vinh-Hung, V, Burzykowski, T, Van de Steene, J, et al. Post-surgery Radiation in Early Breast Cancer: Survival Analysis of Registry Data. Radiotherapy Oncology 64:281–90. 2002.
5. Adjuvant Therapy for Breast Cancer. NIH Consensus Statement. Online 2000 November 1–3; 17:1–23.
6. Woodward, WA. Radiation Reduces Risk of Recurrence in Node-Positive Mastectomy Patients. Presented at the American Society for Therapeutic Radiology and Oncology. 44th Annual Meeting. Houston, TX. Oct. 8, 2002.
7. Fisher, B, et al. Lumpectomy and Radiation Therapy for the Treatment of Intraductal Breast Cancer: Findings from National Surgical Adjuvant Breast and Bowel Project B-17. Journal of Clinical Oncology 16:441–52. 1998.
8. Keisch, M, Vicini, F, Kuske, RR, et al. Initial Clinical Experience with the MammoSite Breast Brachytherapy Applicator in Women with Early-stage Breast Cancer Treated with Breast-conserving Therapy. International Journal of Radiation Oncology, Biology, Physics 55:289–93. 2003.

9. Vicini, FA, Baglan, KL, Kestin, LL, et al. Accelerated Treatment of Breast Cancer. Journal of Clinical Oncology 19:1993–2001, 2001.

10. Adjuvant Therapy for Breast Cancer. Op cit.

11. Leonard, RCF, Lind, M, Twelves, C, et al. Conventional Adjuvant Chemotherapy versus Single-Cycle, Autograft-supported, High-dose, Late-intensification Chemotherapy in High-Risk Breast Cancer Patients: A Randomized Trial. Journal of the National Cancer Institute 96:1076–83. 2004.

12. Hormones in Breast Cancer Treatment. http://www.breastcancer.org.

13. National Surgical Adjuvant Breast and Bowel Project. www.nsabp.pitt.edu.

14. Ibid.

15. Punglia, S, Kuntz, KM, Lee, JH, et al. Radiation Therapy Plus Tamoxifen versus Tamoxifen Alone After Breast-conserving Surgery in Postmenopausal Women with Stage 1 Breast Cancer: A Decision Analysis. Journal of Clinical Oncology 21:2260–67. 2003.

16. National Surgical Adjuvant Breast and Bowel Project. Op cit.

17. Longer-Term Data Confirm Raloxifene Reduces the Risk of Breast Cancer in Older Women. Clinical Trial Results. National Cancer Institute. www.cancer.gov/clinicaltrials/results/raloxifene0604.

18. Chung, CT, Carlson, RW. The Role of Armoatase Inhibitors in Early Breast Cancer. Current Treatment Options in Oncology 4:133–40. 2003.

19. The ATAC (Arimidex, Tamoxifen, Alone or in Combination) Adjuvant Breast Cancer Trial in Postmenopausal Patients: Factors Influencing the Success of Patient Recruitment. European Journal of Cancer 38:1984–86. 2002.

20. Goss, PE, Ingle, JN, Martino, S, et al. A Randomized Trial of Letrozole in Postmenopausal Women After 5 Years of Tamoxifen Therapy for Early Stage Breast Cancer. New England Journal of Medicine 349:1793–1801. 2003.

21. Slamon, DJ, Leyand-Jones, B, Shak, S, et al. Use of Chemotherapy Plus a Monoclonal Antibody Against HERR2 for Metastatic Breast Cancer that Overexpresses HER2. New England Journal of Medicine 344:783–92. 2001.

22. Ibid.

23. Stadtmauer, EA, O'Neill, A, Goldstein, LJ, et al. Conventional-Dose Chemotherapy Compared with High-Dose Chemotherapy plus Autologous Hematopoietic Stem-Cell Transplantation for Metastatic Breast Cancer. New England Journal of Medicine 342:1069–76. 2000.

## CHAPTER 4

1. Newman, LA, Kuerer, HM, Hunt, KK, et al. Educational Review: Role of the Surgeon in Hereditary Breast Cancer. Annals of Surgical Oncology 8:368–78. 2001.

2. Scheuer, L, Kauff, N, Robson, M, et al. Outcome of Preventive Surgery and Screening for Breast and Ovarian Cancer in BRCA Mutation Carriers. Journal of Clinical Oncology 20:1260–68. 2002.

3. Burke, W, Atkins, D, Gwinn, M, et al. Genetic Test Evaluation: Information Needs of Clinicians, Policy Makers, and the Public. American Journal of Epidemiology 156:311–18. 2002.

## CHAPTER 5

1. Roentgen and the Discovery of Xrays. www.xray.hmc.psu.edu.

2. Advances in Mammography and Breast Imagining. www.sys.uea.ac.uk.

3. History of the Mammography. www.gehealthcare.com/rad.

4. Ballard-Barbash, R. Breast Cancer Surveillance Consortium: A National Mammography Screening and Outcomes Database. American Journal of Radiology 169:1001–8. 1997.

5. Mammography Quality Standards Act. www.fda.gov/cdrh/mammography.

6. Shapiro, S. Periodic Screening for Breast Cancer: The HIP Randomized Controlled Trial Health Insurance Plan. Journal National Cancer Institute Monograph 22:27–30. 1997; Shapiro, S, Venet, W, Strax, P, et al. Periodic Screening for Breast Cancer: The Health Insurance Plan Project and Its Sequelae, 1963–1986. Baltimore: Johns Hopkins University Press. 1988.

7. Report of the Working Group to Review the National Cancer Institute-American Cancer Society Breast Cancer Detection Demonstration Project. Journal of the National Cancer Institute 62:639–709. 1979.

8. Smart, CA, Byrne, CA, Smith, RA. Twenty-Year Follow Up of the Breast Cancers Diagnosed during the Breast Cancer Detection Demonstration Project. CA Cancer Journal for Clinicians 47:134–49. 1997.

9. Seidman, H, Gleb, SK, Silverberg, E, et al. Survival Experience in the Breast Cancer Detection Demonstration Project. CA 37:258–90. 1987.

10. Ibid.

11. Michaelson, J, Lebovic, G. Women Ignoring Message About Mammograms. Cancer Online. June 21, 2004.

12. Ballard-Barbash, B. Op cit.

13. Mushlin, AI, Kouides, RW, Shapiro, DE. Estimating the Accuracy of Screening Mammography: A Meta-Analysis. American Journal of Preventive Medicine 14:143–53. 1998; Humphrey, LL, Helfand, M, Chan, BKS. Breast Cancer Screening: A Summary of the Evidence for the U.S. Preventive Services Task Force. Annals Internal Medicine 137:347–60. 2002.

14. Kleit, AN, Ruiz, JF. False Positive Mammograms and Detection Controlled Estimation. Health Services Research 38:1207–28. 2003.

15. Beam, CA, Layde, PM, Sullivan, DC. Variability in the Interpretation of Screening Mammograms by US Radiologists. Findings from a National Sample. Archives of Internal Medicine 156:209–13. 1996.

16. Esserman, L, Cowley, CE, Kirkpatrick, A, et al. Improving the Accuracy of Mammography: Volume and Outcome Relationships. Journal of the National Cancer Institute 94:369–74. 2002.

17. Food and Drug Administration. US Dept of Health and Human Services. Federal Register. Quality Mammography Standards; Final Rule. 21 CFR Parts 16 and 900. Oct 28, 1997. p. 55852; National Health Service (NHS) Breast Screening Radiologists Quality Assurance Committee. Quality Assurance Guidelines for Radiologists. National Health Service Breast Screening Programme. Publ No. 15. Sheffield (UK): NHSBSP Publications. Revised May 1997.

18. Smith-Bindman, R, Chu, PW, Miglioretti, DL, et al. Comparison of Screening Mammography in the United States and the United Kingdom. Journal of the American Medical Association. 290:2129–37. 2003.

19. Elmore, JG, Miglioretti, DL, Carney, PA. Does Practice Make Perfect When Interpreting Mammography? Part II. Journal of the National Cancer Institute 95:250–52. 2003.

20. Elmore, JG, Barton, MB, Moceri, VM, et al. Ten-Year Risk of False Positive Screening Mammograms and Clinical Breast Examinations. New England Journal of Medicine 338:1089–96. 1998.

21. Kerlikowske, K, Barclay, J. Outcomes of Modern Screening Mammography. Journal of the National Cancer Institute Monographs 22:105–11. 1997.

22. Banks, E, Reeves, G, Beral, V, et al. Impact of the Use of Hormone Replacement Therapy on False Positive Recall in the NHS Breast Screening Programme: Results from the Million Women Study. British Medical Journal 328:1291–92. 2004.

23. Burnside, E, Belkora, JK, Esserman, LJ. The Impact of Alternative Practices on the Cost and Quality of Mammographic Screening in the United States. Clinical Breast Cancer 2:145–52. 2001.

24. Zahl, PH, Strand, BH, Maehlen, J. Incidence of Breast Cancer in Norway and Sweden during Introduction of Nationwide Screening: Prospective Cohort Study. British Medical Journal 328:921–24. 2004.

25. Improving Methods for Breast Cancer Detection and Diagnosis. National Cancer Institute Cancer Facts. April 26, 2002.

26. Ibid.

27. Ibid.

28. Kriege, M, Brekelmans, CTM, Boetes, C, et al. Efficacy of MRI and Mammography for Breast Cancer Screening in Women with a Familial or Genetic Predisposition. New England Journal of Medicine 351:427–37. 2004.

29. Improving Methods for Breast Cancer Detection and Diagnosis. National Cancer Institute Cancer Facts. Op cit.

30. Vargas, HI, Agbunag, RV, Kalinowski, A, et al. The Clinical Utility of Tc-99m Sestamibi Scintimammography in Detecting Multicentric Breast Cancer. The American Surgeon 67:1204–8. 2001.

31. Lumachi, F, Ferretti, G, Povolato, M, et al. Accuracy of Technetium-99m Sestamibi Scintimammography and X-ray Mammography in Premenopausal Women with Suspected Breast Cancer. European Journal of Nuclear Medicine 28:1776–79. 2001; Danielsson, R, Reihner, E, Grabowska, A, et al. The Role of Scintimammography with 99m Tc-Sestamibi as a Complementary Diagnostic Technique in the detection of Breast Cancer. Acta Radiologica 41:441–45. 2000.

32. Khalkhali, I, Villanueva-Meyer, J, Edell, SL, et al. Diagnostic Accuracy of 99mTc-Sestamibi Breast Imaging: Multicenter Trial Results. Journal of Nuclear Medicine 41:1973–79. 2000.

33. Improving Methods for Breast Cancer Detection and Diagnosis. National Cancer Institute Cancer Facts. Op cit.

34. Keyserlingk, J. Time to Reassess the Value of Infrared Breast Imaging? Oncology News Int. Vol 6, No. 9. 1997.

35. Breast Thermography. International Academy of Clinical Thermology. www.iact.org.

36. Improving Methods for Breast Cancer Detection and Diagnosis. National Cancer Institute Cancer Facts. Op cit.

37. Ibid.

38. Dooley, WC, Ljung, BM, Veronesi, U, et al. Ductal Lavage for Detection of Cellular Atypia in Women at High Risk for Breast Cancer. Journal of the National Cancer Institute 93:1624–31. 2001.

39. Dooley, WC. Endoscopic Visualization of Breast Tumors. Journal of the American Medical Association 284:1518. 2000.

40. Barton, MB, Harris, R, Fletcher, SW. Does this Patient Have Breast Cancer: The Screening Clinical Examination: Should It Be Done? How? Journal of the American Medical Association 282:1270–80. 1999.

## CHAPTER 6

1. Shapiro, S, Venet, W, Strax, P, et al. Periodic Screening for Breast Cancer: The Health Insurance Plan Project and Tits Sequelae, 1963–1983. Baltimore: Johns Hopkins University Press. 1988; Shapiro, S, Venet, W, Strax, P, et al. Periodic Screening for Breast Cancer: The HIP Randomized Controlled

Trial Health Insurance Plan. Journal of the National Cancer Institite Monograph 22:27–30. 1997.

2. Andersson, I, Aspegren, K. Janzon, L., et al. Mammographic Screening and Mortality from Breast Cancer: The Malmo Mammographic Screening Trial. British Medical Journal 297:943–48. 1988.

3. Roberts, MM, Alexander, FE, Anderson, TJ, et al. Edinburgh Trial of Screening for Breast Cancer: Mortality at Seven Years. Lancet 335:241–46. 1990; Alexander, FE, Anderson, TJ, Brown, HK, et al. The Edinburgh Randomized Trial of Breast Cancer Screening. British Journal of Cancer 70:542–48.1994.

4. Miller, AB, Baines, CJ, To, T, el al. Canadian National Breast Screening Study: 1. Breast Cancer Detection and Death Rates among Women Aged 40–49 Years. Canadian Medical Association Journal 147:1459–76. 1992.

5. Miller, AB, Baines, CJ, To, T, et al. Canadian National Breast Screening Study: 2. Breast Cancer Detection and Death Rates Among Women Aged 50–59 Years. Canadian Medical Association Journal 147:1477–88. 1992.

6. Frisell, J, Lidbrink, E, Hellstrom, L, et al. Followup after 11 Years: Update of Mortality Results in the Stockholm Mammographic Screening Trial. Breast Cancer Research and Treatment 45:263–70. 1997.

7. Bjurstam, N, Bjorneld, L, Duffy, SW, et al. The Gothenburg Breast Screening Trial: First Results on Mortality, Incidence, and Mode of Detection for Women Ages 39–49 Years at Randomization. Cancer 80:2091–99. 1997.

8. Tabar, L, Fagerberg, G, Duffy SE, et al. The Swedish Two County Trial of Mammographic Screening for Breast Cancer: Recent Results and Calculation of Benefit. Journal of Epidemiology Community Health 43:107–14. 1989; Tabar, L, Fagerberg, G, Duffy, SW, et al. Update of the Swedish Two-County Program of Mammographic Screening for Breast Cancer. Radiology Clinics of North America 30:187–210. 1992.

9. Seidman, H, Gelb, SK, Silverberg, E, et al. Survival Experience in the Breast Cancer Detection Demonstration Project. CA Cancer Journal for Clinicians 37:258–90. 1987.

10. Tabar, L, Vitak, B, Chen, HHT, et al. Beyond Tandomized Controlled Trials: Organized Mammographic Screening Substantially Reduces Breast Carcinoma Mortality. Cancer 91:1724–31. 2001.

11. Miller, AM, To, T, Baines, CJ, et al. Canadian National Breast Screening Study-2: 13 Years Result of a Randomized Trial in Women aged 50–59 Years. Journal of the National Cancer Institute 92:1490–99. 2000.

# CHAPTER 7

1. Harris, R, Leininger, L. Clinical Strategies for Breast Cancer Screening: Weighing and Using the Evidence. Annals of Internal Medicine 122:539–47. 1995.

2. Berry, DA. Benefits and Risks of Screening Mammogram for Women in Their Forties: A Statistical Appraisal. Journal of the National Cancer Institute 90:1431–39. 1998; Kerlikowske, K. Efficacy of Screening Mammography Among Women Aged 40–49 Years and 50 to 69 Years: Comparison of Relative and Absolute Benefit. Journal of the National Cancer Institute Monographs 22:79–86. 1997.

3. Gotzsche, PC, Olsen, O. Is Screening for Breast Cancer with Mammography Justifiable? Lancet 355:129–34. 2000.

4. Horton, R. Screening Mammography—An Overview Revisited. Lancet 358:1284–85. 2001.

5. Olsen, O, Gotzsche, PC. Cochrane Review on Screening for Breast Cancer with Mammography. Lancet 358:1340–42. 2001.

6. Tabar, L, Yen, MF, Vitak, B, et al. Mammography Service Screening and Mortality in Breast Cancer Patients: 20-Year Follow Up Before and After Introduction of Screening. Lancet 361:1405–10. 2003.

7. Seidman, H, Gelb, SK, Silverberg, E, et al. Survival Experience in the Breast Cancer Detection Demonstration Project. CA Cancer Journal for Clinicians 37:258–90. 1987.

8. Miller, AB, To, T, Baines, CJ, et al. The Canadian National Breast Screening Study-1: Breast Cancer Mortality after 11 to 16 Years of Follow Up: A Randomized Screening Trial of Mammography in Women Age 40 to 49 Years. Annals of Internal Medicine 137:305–12. 2002.

9. Gelmon, KA, Olivotto, I. The Mammography Screening Debate: Time to Move On. Lancet 359:904–5. 2002.

10. Nystrom, L, Andersson, I, Bjurstam, N, et al. Long-term Effects of Mammography Screening: Updated Overview of the Swedish Randomised Trials. Lancet 359:909–19. 2002.

11. Gelmon, KA, Olivotto, I. Op. cit.

12. Karras, T. The Mammogram Screening Controversy: When Should You Start? CNN.com. Sept. 27, 1999.

13. Irwig, L, Barratt, A, Salkeld, G. Review of the Evidence About the Value of Mammographic Screening in 40–49 Year Old Women. Sydney, Australia: NHMRC National Breast Cancer Centre. 1997.

14. National Institutes of Health. Consensus Development Consensus Statement: Breast Cancer Screening for Women Ages 40–49. Bethesda, MD: National Institutes of Health. January 1997.

15. Mandelblatt, J, Saha, S, Teutsch, S, et al. The Cost-Effectiveness of Screening Mammography Beyond Age 65. Annals of Internal Medicine 139:835–42. 2003.

16. Barratt, A, Irwig, L, Glasziou, P, et al. Benefits, Harms and Costs of Screening Mammography in Women 70 Years and Over: A Systematic Review. Medical Journal of Australia 176:266–71. 2002.

17. Leitch, AM, Dodd, GD, Costanza, M, et al. American Cancer Society Guidelines for the Early Detection of Beast Cancer: Update 1997. CA Cancer Journal for Clinicians 47:150–3. 1997.

18. Kerlikowske, K, Salzmann, P, Phillips, KA, et al. Continuing Screening Mammography in Women Aged 70 to 79 Years: Impact on Life Expectancy and Cost-effectiveness. Journal of the American Medical Association 282:2156–63. 1999.

19. Jones, BA, Patterson, EA, Calvocoressi, L, et al. Mammography Screening in African American Women. Cancer 97:258–72. 2002.

20. Thornston, H, Edwards, A, Baum, M. Women Need Better Information about Routine Mammography. British Medical Journal 327:101–3. 2003.

21. Gigerenzer, G. Reckoning with Risk. London: Penguin. 2002.

22. Croft, E, Barratt, A, Butow, P. Information about Tests for Breast Cancer: What Are We Telling People. Journal of Family Practice 51:858–60. 2002.

23. Jorgensen, KJ, Gotzsche, PC. Presentation on Websites of Possible Benefits and Harms from Screening for Breast Cancer: Cross Sectional Study. British Medical Journal 328:148–51. 2004.

24. Cancer Prevention and Early Detection Facts and Figures 2003. American Cancer Society. 2003.

25. Humphrey, LL, Helfand, M, Chan, BKS, et al. Breast Cancer Screening: A Summary of the Evidence for the U.S. Preventive Services Task Force. Annals of Internal Medicine 137:347–60. 2002.

26. NCI Statement on Mammography. National Cancer Institute New Center. February 21, 2002.

27. Screening for Breast Cancer: Recommendations and Rationale. US Preventive Services Task Force. Annals of Internal Medicine 137:344–46. 2003.

## CHAPTER 8

1. Stewart, MA. Effective Physician-Patient Communication and Health Outcomes: A Review. Canadian Medical Association Journal 152:1423–33. 1996.

2. Roter, DL, Hall, JA, Aoki, Y. Physician Gender Effects in Medical Communication: A Meta-Analytic Review. Journal of the American Medical Association 288:756–64. 2002.

3. Bakker, DA, Fitch, MI, Gray, R, et al. Patient–Health Care Provider Communication during Chemotherapy Treatment: The Perspectives of Women with Breast Cancer. Patient Education Counseling 43:61–71. 2001.

4. Lerman, C, Daly, M, Walsh, WP, et al. Communication between Patients with Breast Cancer and Health Care Providers. Determinants and Implications. Cancer 72:2612–20. 1992.

5. Blanchard, CG, Labrecque, MS, Ruckdeschel, JC, et al. Information and Decision-Making Preferences of Hospitalized Adult Cancer Patients. Social Science and Medicine 27:1139–45. 1988.

6. Lerman, C, et al. Op cit.

7. Rabinowitz, B. Understanding and Intervening in Breast Cancer's Emotional and Sexual Side Effects. Current Womens Health Rep 2:140–7. 2002.

8. Alder, J, Bitzer, J. Retrospective Evaluation of the Treatment for Breast Cancer: How Does the Patient's Personal Experience of the Treatment Affect Later Adjustment to the Illness? Archives Women Mental Health 6:91–97. 2003.

9. McWilliam, CL, Brown, JB, Steward, M. Breast Cancer Patients' Experiences of Patient-Doctor Communication: A Working Relationship. Patient Education Counseling 39:191–204. 2000.

10. Lerman, C, et al. Op cit.

11. Paling, J. Strategies to Help Patients Understand Risks. British Medical Journal 327:745–48. 2003.

12. Lloyd, A, Hayes, P, Bell, RF, et al. The Role of Risk and Benefit Perception in Informed Consent for Surgery. Medical Decision Making 21:141–49. 2001.

13. Navon, L. Cultural Views of Cancer Around the World. Cancer Nursing 22:39–45. 1999.

14. Dey, P, Bundred, N, Gibbs, A, et al. Costs and Benefits of a One Stop Clinic Compared with a Dedicated Breast Clinic: Randomised Controlled Trial. British Medical Journal 324:507. 2002.

15. Aachariae, R, Pedersen, CG, Jensen, AB, et al. Association of Perceived Physician Communication Style with Patient Satisfaction, Distress, Cancer-related Self-efficacy, and Perceived Control Over the Disease. British Journal of Cancer 88:658–65. 2003.

16. Cegala, DJ, Lenzmeier, BS. Physician Communication Skills Training: A Review of Theoretical Backgrounds, Objectives, and Skills. Medical Education 36:1004–16. 2002.

17. Katz, J. The Silent World of the Doctor and Patient. New York: The Free Press. 1984.

18. Brown, JB, Stewart, M, McWilliam, CL. Using the Patient-centered Method to Achieve Excellence in Care for Women with Breast Cancer. Patient Education Counseling 38:121–29. 1999.
19. Degner, LF, Kristjanson, LJ, Bowman, D, et al. Information Needs and Decisional Preferences in Women with Breast Cancer. Journal of the American Medical Association 277:1485–92. 1997.
20. Dowsett, SM, Saul, JL, Butow, PN, et al. Communication Styles in the Cancer Consultation: Preferences for a Patient-centered Approach. PsychoOncology 9:147–56. 2000.
21. Beaver, K, Luker, KA, Owens, RG, et al. Treatment Decision Making in Women Newly Diagnosed with Breast Cancer. Cancer Nursing 19:8–19. 1996.
22. Degner, LF, et al. Op cit.
23. Gattellari, M, Butow, PN, Tattersall, MH. Sharing Decisions in Cancer Care. Social Science and Medicine 52:1865–78. 2001.
24. Beckman, HB, Frankel, RM. The Effect of Physician Behavior on the Collection of Data. Annals Internal Medicine 101:692–96. 1984.
25. Lerman, C, et al. Op cit.
26. Ibid.
27. Ong, LM, Visser, MR, Lammes, FB, et al. Effect of Providing Cancer Patients with the Audiotaped Initial Consultation on Satisfaction, Recall, and Quality of Life: A Randomized, Double-blind Study. Journal of Clinical Oncology 18:3052–60. 2000.
28. McConnell, D, Butow, PN, Tattersall, MH. Audiotapes and Letters to Patients: The Practice and Views of Oncologists, Surgeons, and General Practitioners. British Journal of Cancer 79:1782–88. 1999.
29. Scott, JT, Entwistle, VA, Sowden, AJ, et al. Giving Tape Recordings or Written Summaries of Consultations to People with Cancer: A Systematic Review. Health Expectations 4:162–69. 2001.
30. Sepucha, KR, Belkora, JK, Mutchnick, S, et al. Consultation Planning to Help Breast Cancer Patients Prepare for Medical Consultations: Effect on Communication and Satisfaction for Patients and Physicians. Journal of Clinical Oncology 20:2695–2700. 2002.

## CHAPTER 9

1. Holland, JC. Psychological Care of Patients: Psycho-Oncology's Contribution. Journal of Clinical Oncology 23s:253s–65s. 2003. p. 259.
2. Newell, S, Sason-Fisher, RW, Girgis, A, et al. The Physical and Psychosocial Experiences of Patients Attending an Outpatient Medical Oncology

Department: A Cross-sectional Study. European Journal of Cancer Care 8:73–82. 1999.

3. Pascoe, S, Edelman, S, Kidman, A. Prevalence of Psychological Distress and Use of Support Services by Cancer Patients at Sydney Hospitals. Australia New Zealand Journal of Psychiatry 34:785–91. 2000.

4. Stewart, DE, Cheung, AM, Duff, S, et al. Attributions of Cause and Recurrence in Long-Term Breast Cancer Survivors. Psycho Oncology 10:179–83. 2001.

5. McKenna, MC, Zevon, MA, Corn, B, et al. Psychosocial Factors and the Development of Breast Cancer: A Meta Analysis. Health Psychology 18:520–31. 1999.

6. Greer, S, Morris, T, Pettigale, KW. Psychological Response to Breast Cancer; Effect on Outcome. Lancet ii:785–87. 1979; Levy, SM, Lee, J, Bagley, C, et al. Survival Hazards Analysis in First Recurrent Breast Cancer Patients: 7 Year Follow Up. Psychosomatic Medicine 50:520–28. 1988.

7. Jamieson, RN, Burish, TG, Willston, KA. Psychogenic Factor in Predicting Survival of Breast Cancer Patients. Journal of Clinical Oncology 5:768–72. 1987; Buddeberg, C, Wolf, C, Seiber, M, et al. Coping Strategies and Course of Disease of Breast Cancer Patients. Psychotherapy and Psychosomatics 55:151–57. 1991.

8. Watson, M, Haviland, JS, Greer, S, et al. Influence of Psychological Response on Survival in Breast Cancer: A Population Based Cohort Study. Lancet 354:1331–36. 1999.

9. Petticrew, M, Bell, R, Hunter, D. Influence of Psychological Coping on Survival and Recurrence in People with Cancer: Systematic Review. British Medical Journal 325:1066–66. 2002.

10. Butow, P. 1996. Op cit.

11. Marlow, B, Cartmill, T, Cieplucha, H, et al. An Interactive Process Model of Psychosocial Support Needs for Women Living with Breast Cancer. Psycho Oncology 12:319–30. 2003.

12. Shapiro, S, Lopez, A, Schwartz, G, et al. Quality of Life and Breast Cancer: Relationship of Psychosocial Variables. Journal of Clinical Psychology 57:501–19. 2001.

13. Figueiredo, MI, Fries, E, Ingram, KM. The Role of Disclosure Patterns and Unsupportive Social Interactions in the Well-Being of Breast Cancer Patients. Psycho Oncology 13:96–105. 2004.

14. Meyer, T, Mark, M. Effects of Psychosocial Interventions with Adult Cancer Patients: A Meta Analysis of Randomized Experiments. Health Psychology 14:101–8. 1995.

15. Parker, PA, Baile, WF, DeMoor, C, et al. Psychosocial and Demographic Predictors of Quality of Life in a Large Sample of Cancer Patients. Psycho Oncology 12:193–93. 2003.
16. Thewes, B, Meiser, B, Richard, J, et al. The Fertility and Menopause Related Information Needs of Younger Women with a Diagnosis of Breast Cancer: A Qualitative Study. Psycho Oncology 12:500–11. 2003.
17. Ganz, P. Menopause and Breast Cancer: Symptoms, Late Effects and Their Management. Seminars in Oncology 28:274–83. 2001.
18. Ganz, P, Rowland, J, Desmond, K, et al. Life After Breast Cancer: Understanding Women's Health-Related Quality of Life and Sexual Functioning. Journal of Clinical Oncology 16:501–14. 1998.
19. Redman, S, Turner, J, Davis, C. Improving Supportive Care for Women with Breast Cancer in Australia: The Challenge of Modifying Health Systems. Psycho-Oncology 12:521–31. 2003.
20. Butow, P, Kazemi, J, Beeney, L, et al. When the Diagnosis is Cancer: Patient Communication Experiences and Preferences. Cancer 77:2630–7. 1996; Butow, P, Maclean, M, Dunn, S, et al. The Dynamics of Change: Cancer Patients' Preferences for Information, Involvement, and Support. Annals of Oncology 8:857–63. 1997; Butow, P, Brown, R, Cogar, S, et al. Oncologists' Reactions to Cancer Patients' Verbal Cues. Psycho-Oncology 11:47–58. 2002.
21. Butow, P, et al. 1996. Op cit.
22. Maquire, P, Faulkner, A, Booth, K, et al. Helping Cancer Patients Disclose Their Concerns. European Journal of Cancer 32A:78–81. 1996.
23. Brown, RF, Dunn, S, Butow, P. Meeting Patient Expectations in the Cancer Consultation. Annals of Oncology 8:877–82. 1997.
24. Holland, JC (ed.). Psycho Oncology. New York: Oxford University Press. 1998.
25. National Comprehensive Cancer Network (NCCN): Distress Management Clinical Practice Guidelines. Journal of the National Comprehensive Cancer Network 1:344–74. 2003.

# Index

## ABOUT THE AUTHOR

MADELON L. FINKEL, Ph.D., is Professor of Clinical Public Health at the Weill Medical College of Cornell University. She serves as Director of Cornell Analytic Consulting Services, and Director of the Office of International Medical Education at Weill Medical College. Her research has been focused on women's health issues, including studies of teenage sexual behavior and also hormone replacement therapy. Finkel has been honored with the Excellence in Teaching Award at Weill Medical College, where she has taught for more than two decades.